Pocket Guide
to Critical Care
Pharmacotherapy

Pocket Guide to Critical Care Pharmacotherapy

By

John Papadopoulos, BS, PharmD, FCCM, BCNSP

Associate Professor of Pharmacy Practice
Arnold & Marie Schwartz College
of Pharmacy and Health Sciences
Brooklyn, New York
and
Critical Care Pharmacist
Clinical Instructor of Medicine
Department of Medicine
New York University Medical Center
New York, New York

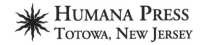

HUMANA PRESS
TOTOWA, NEW JERSEY

Due diligence has been taken by the publishers, editors, and authors of this book to assure the accuracy of the information published and to describe generally accepted practices. The contributors herein have carefully checked to ensure that the drug selections and dosages set forth in this text are accurate and in accord with the standards accepted at the time of publication. Notwithstanding, as new research, changes in government regulations, and knowledge from clinical experience relating to drug therapy and drug reactions constantly occurs, the reader is advised to check the product information provided by the manufacturer of each drug for any change in dosages or for additional warnings and contraindications. This is of utmost importance when the recommended drug herein is a new or infrequently used drug. It is the responsibility of the treating physician to determine dosages and treatment strategies for individual patients. Further it is the responsibility of the health care provider to ascertain the Food and Drug Administration status of each drug or device used in their clinical practice. The publisher, editors, and authors are not responsible for errors or omissions or for any consequences from the application of the information presented in this book and make no warranty, express or implied, with respect to the contents in this publication.

This publication is printed on acid-free paper. ∞
ANSI Z39.48-1984 (American Standards Institute) Permanence of Paper for Printed Library Materials.

Cover design by Karen Schulz

Production Editor: Amy Thau

For additional copies, pricing for bulk purchases, and/or information about other Humana titles, contact Humana at the above address or at any of the following numbers: Tel.: 1-800-SPRINGER; Fax: 973-256-8314; or visit our Website: http://humanapress.com

Photocopy Authorization Policy:

Printed in the United States of America. 10 9 8 7 6 5 4 3 2 1
eISBN 13: 978-1-59745-488-9
Library of Congress Control Number: 2007938421

*This handbook is dedicated to my wife Maria,
my children, Theodore Thomas and Eleni Thalia, and
my mother Eleni. I am grateful for your collective
understanding of my professional commitment.*

Preface

Critical care medicine is a cutting-edge medical field that is highly evidence-based. Studies are continuously published that alter the approach to patient care. As a critical care clinician, I am aware of the tremendous commitment required to provide optimal evidence-based care. *Pocket Guide to Critical Care Pharmacotherapy* covers the most common ailments observed in adult critically-ill patients. I utilize an algorithmic, easy-to-follow, systematic approach. Additionally, I provide references and web links for many disease states, for clinicians who want to review the available literature in greater detail.

The contents of this handbook should be utilized as a guide and in addition to sound clinical judgment. Consult full prescribing information and take into consideration each drug's pharmacokinetic profile, contraindications, warnings, precautions, adverse reactions, potential drug interactions, and monitoring parameters before use.

Every effort was made to ensure the accuracy of *Pocket Guide to Critical Care Pharmacotherapy*. The author, editor, and publisher are not responsible for errors or omissions or for any consequences associated with the utilization of the contents of this handbook.

John Papadopoulos, BS, PharmD, FCCM, BCNSP

Contents

Preface vii
Editor xi
List of Tables xiii

1. Advance Cardiac Life Support 1
2. Cardiovascular 21
3. Cerebrovascular 55
4. Critical Care 65
5. Dermatology 101
6. Endocrinology 103
7. Gastrointestinal 109
8. Hematology 119
9. Infectious Disease 125
10. Neurology 131
11. Nutrition 137
12. Psychiatric Disorders 143
13. Pulmonary 149
14. Renal 155

Index 183

Editor

David R. Schwartz, MD • Section Chief, Critical Care
Medicine, Assistant Professor of Medicine,
Department of Medicine, New York University
Medical Center, New York, New York

List of Tables

Chapter 1

1.1. ACLS Pulseless Arrest Algorithm

1.2. Ventricular Fibrillation/Pulseless Ventricular Tachycardia Algorithm

1.3. Pulseless Electrical Activity Algorithm

1.4. Asystole Algorithm

1.5. Bradycardia Algorithm (slow [HR <60 bpm] or Relatively Slow)

1.6. Tachycardia Algorithm Overview

1.7. Management of Stable Atrial Fibrillation/ Atrial Flutter

1.8. Management of Narrow Complex Stable Supraventricular Tachycardia (QRS < 0.12 s)

1.9. Management of Stable Ventricular Tachycardia

1.10. Synchronized Cardioversion Algorithm for the Management of Symptomatic Tachycardia

1.11. Common Drugs Utilized During ACLS

1.12. Pulseless Electrical Activity: *Causes (HATCH HMO pH) and Management*

1.13. Pharmacological Management of Anaphylaxis/Anaphylactoid Reactions

Chapter 2

2.1. Thrombolysis in Myocardial Infarction (TIMI) Grade Flows

2.2. TIMI Risk Score

2.3. Short-Term Risk of Death of Nonfatal Myocardial Infarction in Patients Presenting with Unstable Angina (Note: Low-Risk Omitted)

2.4. Acute Pharmacological Management of Unstable Angina and Non-ST Elevation Myocardial Infarction

2.5. Acute Pharmacological Management of ST-Elevation Myocardial Infarction (Non-Invasive or Conservative Strategy)

2.6. Considerations in Patients with Right Ventricular Infarctions

2.7. Contraindications to Fibrinolytic Therapy in Patients with ST-Elevation Myocardial Infarction

2.8. Management of Acute Decompensated Heart Failure

2.9. Vaughan Williams Classification of Antiarrhythmics

2.10. Antithrombotic Pharmacotherapy for Patients with Various Diseases

2.11. Causes and Management of Acquired Torsades de Pointes

2.12. Hypertensive Crises

2.13. Management of Catecholamine Extravasation

2.14. Prevention of Venous Thromboembolism in the ICU Patient

2.15. Management of Deep-Vein Thrombosis and Pulmonary Embolism
2.16. Management of Elevated INRs in Patients Receiving Warfarin Pharmacotherapy

Chapter 3

3.1. General Supportive Care for Patients with an Acute Cerebrovascular Accident
3.2. Blood Pressure Management in the Setting of an Acute Cerebrovascular Accident
3.3. Alteplase Inclusion and Exclusion Criteria for CVA Indication
3.4. Modified National Institute of Health Stroke Scale
3.5. Alteplase Administration Protocol for CVA Indication
3.6. Management of an Alteplase-Induced Intracranial Hemorrhage
3.7. Management of Intracranial Hypertension (ICP $\geq$ 20 mmHg)

Chapter 4

4.1. General Drug Utilization Principles in ICU Care
4.2. Management of Severe Sepsis and Septic Shock
4.3. Sedation, Analgesia, and Delirium Guidelines
4.4. Modified Ramsey Sedation Scale
4.5. Riker Sedation-Agitation Scale
4.6. Confusion Assessment Method for the Diagnosis of Delirium in ICU Patients
4.7. Neuromuscular Blocker Use in the Intensive Care Unit

4.8. Reversal of Nondepolarizing Neuromuscular Blockers

4.9. Factors that Alter the Effects of Neuromuscular Blockers

4.10. Management of Malignant Hyperthermia

4.11. Use of Packed Red Blood Cell Transfusions and Erythropoietin in Critically-Ill Patients

4.12. Propylene Glycol Content of Commonly Utilized Intravenous Medications

4.13. Drug-Induced Fever

4.14. Pharmaceutical Dosage Forms That Should Not Be Crushed

4.15. Stress-Related Mucosal Damage Prophylaxis Protocol

4.16. Therapeutic Drug Monitoring

4.17. Select Antidotes for Toxicological Emergencies

Chapter 5

5.1. Drug-Induced Dermatological Reactions

Chapter 6

6.1. Management of Diabetic Ketoacidosis

6.2. Management of Hyperglycemic Hyperosmolar Nonketotic Syndrome

6.3. Management of Thyrotoxic Crisis and Myxedema Coma

Chapter 7

7.1. Management of Acute Nonvariceal Upper Gastrointestinal Bleeding

7.2. Causes of Diarrhea in the Intensive Care Unit Patient

7.3. Managing the Complications of Cirrhosis

7.4. Drug-Induced Hepatotoxicity
7.5. Drug-Induced Pancreatitis

Chapter 8

8.1. Drug-Induced Hematological Disorders
8.2. Management of Heparin-Induced Thrombocytopenia
8.3. Management of Methemoglobinemia

Chapter 9

9.1. Common Causes of Fever in ICU Patients
9.2. Prevention of Hospital-Acquired and Ventilator-Associated Pneumonia
9.3. Management of Hospital-Acquired and Ventilator-Associated Pneumonia
9.4. Clinical Pulmonary Infection Score Calculation

Chapter 10

10.1. Management of Convulsive Status Epilepticus
10.2. Medications That May Exacerbate Weakness in Myasthenia Gravis

Chapter 11

11.1. Nutrition Assessment
11.2. Principles of Parenteral Nutrition
11.3. Select Drug-Nutrient Interactions
11.4. Strategies to Minimize Aspiration of Gastric Contents during Enteral Nutrition

Chapter 12

12.1. Management of Alcohol Withdrawal
12.2. Management of Serotonin Syndrome

12.3.   Management of Neuroleptic Malignant
        Syndrome

Chapter 13

13.1.   Management of Chronic Obstructive
        Pulmonary Disease
13.2.   Management of Acute Asthma Exacerbations
13.3.   Drug-Induced Pulmonary Diseases

Chapter 14

14.1.   Contrast-Induced Nephropathy Prevention
        Strategy
14.2.   Pharmacological Management of Acute
        Renal Failure
14.3.   Management of Acute Uremic Bleeding
14.4.   Drug-Induced Renal Diseases
14.5.   Management of Acute Hypocalcemia
        (Serum Calcium <8.5 mg/dL)
14.6.   Management of Acute Hypercalcemia
        (Serum Calcium >12 mg/dL)
14.7.   Management of Acute Hypokalemia
        (Serum Potassium <3.5 mEq/L)
14.8.   Management of Acute Hyperkalemia
        (Serum Potassium ≥5.5 mEq/L)
14.9.   Management of Acute Hypomagnesemia
        (Serum Magnesium <1.4 mEq/L)
14.10. Management of Acute Hypermagnesemia
        (Serum Magnesium >2 mEq/L)
14.11. Management of Acute Hyponatremia
        (Serum Sodium <135 mEq/L)
14.12. Management of Acute Hypernatremia
        (Serum Sodium >145 mEq/L)
14.13. Management of Acute Hypophosphatemia
        (<2 mg/dL)

14.14. Management of Hyperphosphatemia (>5 mg/dL)

14.15. Management of Acute Primary Metabolic Acidosis (pH < 7.35)

14.16. Management of Acute Primary Metabolic Alkalosis (pH > 7.45)

14.17. Dosing of Selected Intravenous Anti-Infectives in Patients Receiving Continuous Renal Replacement Therapy

1

Advance Cardiac Life Support

CODE ALGORITHMS

Table 1.1
ACLS Pulseless Arrest Algorithm

- Basic life support (BLS) algorithm → give cardiopulmonary resuscitation (CPR)
  - Push hard and fast (~100 compressions/min)
  - Allow full chest recoil
  - Minimize interruptions in CPR
  - One CPR cycle is equal to 30 compressions then two breaths
    - Five cycles administered every 2 min
    - If possible, compressor should change every 2 min
  - Avoid excessive ventilation leading to unwanted elevation in intrathoracic pressure
  - With advanced airway, give continuous chest compressions without pause for breaths. Administer 8–10 breaths per min and check rhythm every 2 min
- Give oxygen when available
- Attach defibrillator/monitor as soon as possible
- Assess rhythm → shockable rhythm?
  - Shockable ventricular fibrillation/ventricular tachycardia—proceed to Table 1.2
  - Not shockable pulseless electrical activity—proceed to Table 1.3
  - Not shockable asystole—proceed to Table 1.4

Circulation 2005 112(24):IV1–IV203.

From: *Pocket Guide to Critical Care Pharmacotherapy*
By: J. Papadopoulos © Humana Press Inc., Totowa, NJ

Table 1.2
Ventricular Fibrillation/Pulseless Ventricular Tachycardia
Algorithm

- Basic life support (BLS) algorithm → give cardiopulmonary resuscitation (CPR)
- Give one shock
  - Biphasic (device specific): 120–200 J (if unknown use 200 J)
  - Automated external defibrillator (AED) device specific
  - Monophasic: 360 J
- Resume CPR immediately for five cycles every 2 min
- Check rhythm (if shockable, proceed with this algorithm)
- Give one shock as above. Continue CPR while device is charging
- Resume CPR immediately after the shock
- When IV access established, administer vasopressor during CPR (before or after the shock)
  - *Epinephrine* 1 mg intravenous push (IVP), repeat every 3–5 min or *Vasopressin* 40 units IVP × one dose only (replace first or second dose of epinephrine)
- Resume CPR immediately for five cycles
- Check rhythm (if shockable, proceed with this algorithm)
- Give one shock as aforementioned
- Resume CPR immediately after the shock
  - Consider antiarrhythmics (before or after the shock)
    - Amiodarone 300 mg IVP × one dose
      - May administer repeat doses of 150 mg IVP (maximal daily dose equal to 2.2 g)
    - Lidocaine 1–1.5 mg/kg IVP × one dose, then 0.5–0.75 mg/kg IV to a maximum of 3 mg/kg
    - Magnesium 1–2 g IV for torsades de pointes
- Resume CPR immediately for five cycles
- Shock and epinephrine administration as aforementioned every 3–5 min

Table 1.3
Pulseless Electrical Activity Algorithm

- Review most frequent causes (*see* Table 1.12)
- Basic life support (BLS) algorithm → give cardiopulmonary resuscitation (CPR)
  - ○ Concentrate on reversible causes and good CPR
- *Epinephrine* 1 mg intravenous push (IVP), repeat every 3–5 min *or Vasopressin* 40 units IVP × one dose only (replace first or second dose of epinephrine)
- *Atropine* 1 mg IVP (if PEA is *slow*), repeat every 3–5 min as needed to a total of 0.04 mg/kg or three doses

Table 1.4
Asystole Algorithm

- Basic life support (BLS) algorithm → give cardiopulmonary resuscitation (CPR)
  - ○ Concentrate on good CPR
  - ○ Check rhythm every 2 min
  - ○ Check pulse if organized rhythm. Defibrillate if shockable rhythm
- *Epinephrine* 1 mg intravenous push (IVP), repeat every 3–5 min *or Vasopressin* 40 units IVP × one dose only (replace first or second dose of epinephrine)
- Consider *atropine* 1 mg IVP, repeat every 3–5 min as needed to a total of 0.04 mg/kg or three doses

Table 1.5
Bradycardia Algorithm (Slow [Heart Rate <60 bpm] or Relatively Slow)

- Assess airway/breathing/circulation (ABCs)
- Give oxygen
- Establish IV access
- Monitor blood pressure and pulse oximeter

- Obtain and review 12-lead electrocardiogram (ECG)
- Consider causes and differential diagnosis

Serious signs or symptoms owing to bradycardia are present
- *Atropine* 0.5 mg intravenous push (IVP) every 3–5 min up to a total of 0.04 mg/kg or 3 mg
  - Administer every 3 min in severe circumstances
  - Use 1 mg doses in obese patients to avoid paradoxical bradycardia
  - Will not work in denervated transplanted hearts
- Transcutaneous pacing
- *Dopamine* continuous IV infusion 2–10 mcg/kg/min
- *Epinephrine* continuous IV infusion 2–10 mcg/min
- Consider *glucagon* 2–10 mg IV bolus followed by a 2–10 mg/h continuous IV infusion in β-adrenergic blocker or calcium channel blocker-induced bradycardia not responsive to atropine

Serious signs or symptoms of bradycardia are not present
- Type II second-degree or third-degree atriovetricular (AV) block present
  - Prepare for transvenous pacing
  - If symptoms develop, use transcutaneous pacing until transvenous pacing is established
- Type II second-degree or third-degree AV block absent
  - Observe

**Table 1.6
Tachycardia Algorithm Overview**

Evaluate patient
- Assess airway/breathing/circulation (ABCs)
- Give oxygen
- Establish IV access
- Obtain 12-lead electrocardiogram (ECG)
- Identify and treat etiology
- Is the patient stable or unstable?
  - Are there serious signs or symptoms as a result of tachycardia?

Unstable patient (serious signs or symptoms)
- Prepare for immediate cardioversion (*see* Table 1.10)

Stable patient (no serious signs or symptoms as a result of tachycardia)
- *Atrial fibrillation/atrial flutter*
  - Evaluate
    - Cardiac function (i.e., can the patient tolerate negative inotropic medications)
    - Presence of Wolff-Parkinson-White syndrome (WPW)
    - Duration (< or >48 h)
  - *See* atrial fibrillation/atrial flutter algorithm (Table 1.7)
    - Rate control
    - Rhythm control
    - Consider early anticoagulation
- Narrow-complex tachycardias (QRS < 0.12 s)
  - *See* Table 1.8
- Stable wide-complex tachycardia with a regular rhythm
  - If ventricular tachycardia or uncertain rhythm (*see* Table 1.9)
  - If SVT with aberrancy, give adenosine (*see* Table 1.8)
- Stable wide-complex tachycardia with an irregular rhythm
  - If atrial fibrillation with aberrancy (*see* Table 1.7)
  - If atrial fibrillation with WPW (*see* Table 1.7)
  - If polymorphic ventricular tachycardia (*see* Table 1.9)

Table 1.7
Management of Stable Atrial Fibrillation/Atrial Flutter

	Rate control	*Rhythm control (duration ≤ 48 h)*
Normal cardiac function	• β-adrenergic blockers • Diltiazem • Verapamil	• Consider DC cardioversion *or* • Amiodarone • Ibutilide • Flecainide

(Continued)

Table 1.7 *(Continued)*

	Rate control	*Rhythm control (duration ≤ 48 h)*
		• Propafenone • Procainamide
EF < 40%, CHF	• Digoxin • Diltiazem (with caution) • Esmolol (with caution) • Amiodarone	• Consider DC cardioversion *or* • Amiodarone
WPW	• DC cardioversion *or* • Amiodarone • Flecainide • Procainamide • Propafenone • Sotalol	• DC cardioversion *or* • Amiodarone • Flecainide • Procainamide • Propafenone • Sotalol Avoid! • Adenosine • β-adrenergic blockers • Calcium channel blockers • Digoxin

EF, ejection fraction; CHF, chronic heart failure; WPW, Wolff-Parkinson-White syndrome; DC, direct current.

Notes:
Use only one medication initially for rate or rhythm control. Occasionally, two agents may need to be utilized. Combination therapy may cause hypotension, bradycardia, and might be arrhythmogenic.

- Duration of atrial fibrillation/atrial flutter >48 h or unknown.
  - Electrical or chemical cardioversion in a patient without adequate anticoagulation may cause embolization of atrial thrombi.

- o No DC cardioversion if clinically stable.
- o Delay electrical cardioversion.
- o Provided therapeutic anticoagulation for 3 wk, cardiovert *electrically,* then continue therapeutic anticoagulation for four more weeks.
- o Early cardioversion alternative
  - ▪ Begin heparin IV.
  - ▪ Perform transesophageal echocardiogram (TEE) to exclude atrial clot.
  - ▪ If negative, cardiovert *electrically* within 24 h.
  - ▪ Continue therapeutic anticoagulation for 4 wk.

Table 1.8
Management of Narrow Complex Stable Supraventricular Tachycardia (QRS < 0.12 s)

- Attempt therapeutic/diagnostic maneuver if *regular* rhythm. If *irregular* rhythm, proceed to Table 1.7
  - o Vagal stimulation (e.g., carotid massage, valsalva maneuver)
  - o Adenosine 6 mg rapid intravenous push (IVP). If no conversion, give 12 mg rapid IVP may repeat 12 mg dose once
  - o If converts, probably re-entry supraventricular tachycardia (SVT)
  - o If does not convert, probably atrial flutter, ectopic atrial tachycardia, or junctional tachycardia

Paroxysmal (re-entry) supraventricular tachycardia (recurrent/ refractory to vagal stimulation or adenosine)
- Ejection fraction (EF) preserved
  - o Calcium channel blocker
  - o β-adrenergic blocker
  - o Digoxin
  - o Direct current (DC) cardioversion
  - o Consider procainamide, amiodarone, and sotalol
- EF less than 40%, chronic heart failure (CHF)
  - o Digoxin
  - o Amiodarone
  - o Diltiazem (cautious use)
  - o Esmolol (cautious use)

Ectopic or multifocal atrial tachycardia
- EF preserved
  - No DC cardioversion!
  - Calcium channel blocker
  - β-adrenergic blocker
  - Amiodarone
- EF < 40%, CHF
  - No DC cardioversion!
  - Amiodarone
  - Diltiazem (cautious use)
  - Esmolol (cautious use)

Junctional tachycardia
- EF preserved
  - No DC cardioversion!
  - Amiodarone
  - β-adrenergic blocker
  - Calcium channel blocker
- EF < 40%, CHF
  - No DC cardioversion!
  - Amiodarone

Table 1.9
Management of Stable Ventricular Tachycardia

- May go directly to cardioversion if symptomatic or unstable/pulseless
  Monomorphic ventricular tachycardia
- Normal cardiac function
  - Amiodarone
  - Lidocaine
  - Procainamide
  - Sotalol
- Impaired cardiac function (poor ejection fraction)
  - Amiodarone
  - If persistent, use synchronized cardioversion
  Polymorphic ventricular tachycardia
- Use unsynchronized cardioversion if unstable/pulseless

- Normal baseline QT interval and normal cardiac function
  - Treat ischemia
  - Correct electrolyte abnormalities (i.e., hypokalemia and hypomagnesemia)
  - β-adrenergic blockers
  - Lidocaine
  - Amiodarone
  - Procainamide
  - Sotalol
- Normal baseline QT interval and impaired cardiac function (poor ejection fraction)
  - Amiodarone
  - Then use synchronized cardioversion if persistent and stable
- Prolonged baseline QT interval (torsades de pointes?)
  - Correct electrolyte abnormalities (i.e., hypokalemia and hypomagnesemia)
  - Discontinue any medication that can prolong the QT-interval (*see* Table 2.11)
  - Magnesium
  - Overdrive pacing
  - Isoproterenol
  - Lidocaine
  - Synchronized cardioversion if persistant and stable

Table 1.10
Synchronized Cardioversion Algorithm
for the Management of Symptomatic Tachycardia

- If ventricular rate is more than 150 bpm, prepare for immediate cardioversion
  - May administer brief antiarrhythmic trial based on specific arrhythmia
- Immediate cardioversion is generally not needed if ventricular rate is ≤150 bpm

- Consider sedation when possible
  - Diazepam, midazolam, etomidate, barbiturate with or without a narcotic analgesic (e.g., morphine or fentanyl)
- Have bedside access to:
  - Pulse oximeter, IV line, suction device, and intubation equipment
- Synchronized cardioversion
  - For monomorphic ventricular tachycardia, paroxysmal supraventricular tachycardia (SVT), atrial fibrillation, atrial flutter
    - Treat polymorphic ventricular tachycardia (irregular rate and form) as ventricular fibrillation (*see* Table 1.9)
  - Monophasic or (equivalent biphasic) energy dose
    - 100J → 200J → 300J → 360J
      - □ Resynchronize after each cardioversion
      - □ Paroxysmal SVT and atrial flutter often respond to lower energy doses (may start with 50J)
      - □ If delays in synchronization occur and condition is critical, go immediately to unsynchronized shocks

Cardioversion procedure
- Turn on defibrillator
- Attach monitor leads to patient and ensure proper display of patient's rhythm
- Press the "sync" control button to synchronize the defibrillator
  - Look for markers on R waves indicating synchronized mode
  - If needed, adjust monitor gain until synchronized markers occur with each R wave
- Select appropriate energy level
- Position conductor pads on patient or apply gel to paddles
- Position paddles on patient's sternum and apex (apical/posterior position is acceptable)
- Announce to team members "Charging defibrillator—stand clear"
- Press charge button on apex-paddle (right hand)
- When the defibrillator is charged announce to team members
  - "I am going to shock on three."
    - "One—I am clear"

- ■ "Two—you are clear"
- ■ "Three—everybody is clear"
- Apply 25 lbs of pressure if using paddles
- Press the discharge buttons simultaneously and hold until shock delivered
- Check the monitor
- If tachycardia persists, adjust the energy dose according to the algorithm
- Resynchronize after each synchronized cardioversion before repeating above procedure
- To avoid myocardial damage, the interval between shocks should be ≥1 min

Table 1.11
Common Drugs Utilized During ACLS

Drug	Adult dose	Comments
Adenosine	• 6 mg rapid IVP • 12 mg rapid IVP may be administered in 1–2 min if needed • An additional 12 mg rapid IVP may be repeated in 1–2 min if needed	• Follow each dose with a 20 mL IV flush of normal saline • Decrease dose if administered through a central line or concomitant dipyridamole therapy (i.e., 3 mg) • Caffeine and theopylline may antagonize the effect of adenosine
Amiodarone	• *Cardiac arrest:* 300 mg IVP. Additional 150 mg IVP in 3–5 min if needed	• Maximum 24 h dose is 2.2 g

(Continued)

Table 1.11 *(Continued)*

Drug	Adult dose	Comments
	• *SVT/wide-complex tachycardia (stable):* 150 mg IV over 10 min. May repeat 150 mg every 10 min as needed.	• Rapid infusion followed by a continuous IV infusion of 1 mg/min for 6 h, then 0.5 mg/min • Use cautiously with other drugs that prolong the QT-interval • IV diluent (polysorbate 80) may contribute to hypotension • Contains 37.3% iodine by weight • Familiarize yourself with common drug–drug interactions
Atropine	• *Cardiac arrest:* 1 mg IVP every 3–5 min as needed • *Bradycardia:* 0.5–1 mg IVP every 3–5 min	• Maximum dose is 0.04 mg/kg • Dose every 3 min in severe clinical conditions • Doses ≤0.5 mg may cause bradycardia in obese patients. Use 1 mg doses • Use cautiously in the setting of an acute myocardial infarction • Can be given through tracheal tube at 2–2.5 times the recommended dose

(Continued)

Table 1.11 *(Continued)*

Drug	Adult dose	Comments
Digoxin	• Total intravenous loading dose is between 0.5 and 1 mg • Administered as follows: ○ 50% of loading dose initially, followed by 25% every 6 h for two doses • Inject over 1–5 min	• Dose based on ideal body weight • Decrease loading dose in end stage renal disease uncontrolled hypothyroidism, or patients on quinidine by 30–50% • Correct hypokalemia, hypomagnesemia, and hypercalcemia before initiating therapy • May monitor a digoxin level at least 4–6 h after an intravenous loading dose regimen is complete. This may not reflect steady-state concentrations but might be used to assess the adequacy of the loading dose regimen. Digoxin distributes greater into heart tissue than blood; when evaluating any digoxin level, always assess the heart first then the blood

(Continued)

Table 1.11 *(Continued)*

Drug	Adult dose	Comments
		• Digoxin-like immunoreactive substances (found in patients with chronic heart failure, end stage renal disease, liver disease, or third trimester of pregnancy) may cross-react with certain digoxin immunoassays and may result in a false elevation of levels • Familiarize yourself with common drug–drug interactions
Diltiazem	• 0.25 mg/kg IV over 2 min • If response is inadequate after 15 min, may administer 0.35 mg/kg IV over 2 min • May initiate a continuous IV infusion of 5 mg/h. Rate may be increased in 5 mg/h increments up to 15 mg/h if needed	• Hypotension and bradycardia may be seen if combined with a β-adrenergic blocker • Familiarize yourself with common drug–drug interactions
Epinephrine	• *Cardiac arrest:* 1 mg IVP (10 mL of a 1:10,000 solution) every 3–5 min	• High doses may contribute to post-resuscitation myocardial and neurological dysfunction

(Continued)

Table 1.11 *(Continued)*

Drug	Adult dose	Comments
	• *Profound bradycardia:* 2–10 mcg/min continuous IV infusion • *Bronchodilator:* 0.1–0.5 mg SQ (0.1–0.5 mL of a 1: 1000 solution) every 10–15 min until adequate response	• Can be given through tracheal tube at 2–2.5 times the recommended dose • 1:1000 is equal to 1 mg/mL ○ Used for SQ administration • 1:10,000 is equal to 0.1 mg/mL ○ Used for IV administration
Esmolol	• Loading dose: 500 mcg/kg over 1 min • Followed by 50 mcg/kg/min. May increase every 5–10 min by 50 mcg/kg/min increments up to a maximum of 200 mcg/kg/min	• Use cautiously and avoid the loading dose if tenuous hemodynamics • Should be administered through a central line if concentrations greater than 10 mg/mL are utilized • Monitor total volume administered with the continuous IV infusion
Isoproterenol	• 2 mcg/ min continuous IV infusion • Use lower doses in patients who are elderly or have ischemic heart disease (e.g., 0.5 mcg/min)	• Use with extreme caution • Temporary agent for torsades de pointes before transvenous pacing

(Continued)

Table 1.11 *(Continued)*

Drug	*Adult dose*	*Comments*
Lidocaine	• *Cardiac arrest or stable rhythm:* 1–1.5 mg/kg IV. May repeat in 5–10 min with 0.5–0.75 mg/kg IV. May follow bolus with a continuous IV infusion of 1–4 mg/min. If arrhythmia reappears during continuous IV infusion, may bolus with 0.5 mg/kg and reassess	• Maximum dose is 3 mg/kg IV • Decrease continuous IV infusion dose in patients with hepatic or left ventricular dysfunction • Monitor drug levels with prolonged infusions (>24 h) • Can be given through tracheal tube at 2–2.5 times the recommended dose
Magnesium sulfate	• *Cardiac arrest (torsades de pointes):* 1–2 g IVP • *Stable torsades de pointes:* 1–2 g IV over 2–5 min followed by a continuous IV infusion of 0.5–1 g/h	• Use cautiously in patients with renal dysfunction, myasthenia gravis, or concomitant digoxin pharmacotherapy
Sodium bicarbonate	• 1 mEq/kg IVP • Repeat with 0.5 mEq/kg every 10 min as needed	• Not recommended for routine use in cardiac arrest patients • May be useful for cardiac arrest associated with tricyclic antidepressant overdose, hyperkalemic

(Continued)

Table 1.11 *(Continued)*

Drug	Adult dose	Comments
		states, or severe (non-lactic acid) metabolic acidosis • Use arterial blood gases to guide therapy • May increase tissue and central venous acidosis • Complete correction of base deficit should be avoided
Vasopressin	• 40 units IVP (one dose only)	• Metabolic acidosis may not affect vaso-pressin
Verapamil	• 2.5–5 mg IV over 2 min • May administer a second dose of 5–10 mg 15–30 min after the initial dose if inadequate response. Maximum total dose is 20 mg	• Use cautiously in patients with left ven-tricular dysfunction

Circulation 2005 112(24):IV1–IV203.

IVP, intravenous push; SQ, subcutanious; CPR, cardiopulmonary resucitation.

Notes:

1. Pharmacological agents play a secondary role to electric cardiover-sion in unstable patients.
2. Administer intravenous drugs by rapid bolus followed with a 20 mL flush of intravenous fluid and extremity elevation for 10–20 s if peripheral venous access is utilized during resuscitation.

3. Atropine, epinephrine, and lidocaine can be administered through the tracheal tube before venous access is achieved at 2–2.5 times the recommended intravenous dose diluted with 10 mL of normal saline or sterile water. Stop CPR, administer beyond the tip of the endotracheal tube, follow with five quick insufflations to aerosolize the drug, and then resume CPR.
4. All antiarrhythmics can be proarrhythmogenic. Sequential use of more than one agent can result in an adverse drug event. Do not use more than one antiarrhythmic unless absolutely necessary. Electric cardioversion is preferred over a second antiarrhythmic if the initial agent fails.

Table 1.12
Pulseless Electrical Activity: Causes (HATCH HMO pH) and Management

Condition	Evidence	Management
Hypovolemia	Flat neck veins	Intravenous fluids
Acidosis	Arterial blood gases	Sodium bicarbonate, hyperventilation
Tension pneumothorax[a]	History, tracheal deviation, unequal breath sounds, unilateral hyper-resonance to percussion	Needle decompression
Cardiac tamponade[a]	History, emergent bedside echocardiogram results	Pericardiocentesis
Hypoxia	Arterial blood gases, cyanosis, compromised airway	Ventilation, oxygen therapy, positive end expiratory pressure (PEEP)
Hyperkalemia	History, bizarre wide QRS complex, medications	*See* hyperkalemia pathway (Table 14.6)
Myocardial infarction	History, electrocardiogram (ECG), cardiac enzymes	Acute coronary syndrome pathway (Tables 2.4 and 2.5)
Overdose	History, physical exam	Drug specific

(Continued)

Table 1.12 *(Continued)*

Condition	Evidence	Management
Pulmonary embolism[a]	History, emergent bedside echocardiogram results	*See* pulmonary embolism pathway
Hypothermia	Low core body temperature	Raise body temperature

[a]Causes of obstructive shock should be entertained in patients with PEA/asystole with absent or low levels of $ETCO_2$ after placement of invasive airway.

Table 1.13
Pharmacological Management of Anaphylaxis/ Anaphylactoid Reactions

- Stop infusion of culprit drug wherein possible
- Assess airway and cardiopulmonary status
- Place patient in a supine position. Elevate lower extremities if hypotensive
- Administer oxygen at high flow rates if hypoxic (e.g., 6–10 L/min)
- Rapid fluid resuscitation with a crystalloid or a colloid if hypotensive (large volumes may be required)
- Epinephrine
  - Life-threatening situation or in shock: 0.1–0.5 mg IV (1–5 mL of a 1:10,000 solution) over 5 min. May repeat in 5–10 min and as needed or start a continuous IV infusion at 2–10 mcg/min
  - Condition not life-threatening or no vascular access: 0.3–0.5 mg SQ/IM (0.3–0.5 mL of a 1:1000 solution). May repeat in 5–10 min as needed for three total doses
- Antihistamines
  - Diphenhydramine 25–50 mg IV over 5 min q 6 h
- Histamine$_2$-receptor antagonists
  - Famotidine 20 mg IV over 2 min q12h, ranitidine 50 mg IV over 5 min q8h, or cimetidine 300 mg IV over 5 min q6h (must adjust dose of each drug with renal impairment)

- H_2-receptor antagonism without concomitant H_1-receptor antagonism may result in a negative inotropic and chronotropic response
- Hydrocortisone 50–100 mg (or other equivalent dose corticosteroid) IV q6-8h
- If bronchospasm present, use albuterol nebulization 2.5–5 mg every 20 min for 3 doses or racemic epinephrine nebulization 0.5 mL every 3–4 h as needed
  - Epinephrine solution for inhalation—1% (10 mg/mL or 1:100) solution
- If in shock, use norepinephrine or epinephrine continuous IV infusion for hemodynamic support

Cardiovascular

Table 2.1
Thrombolysis in Myocardial Infarction (TIMI)
Grade Flows

TIMI grade	Definition
0	No perfusion; no antegrade flow beyond point of occlusion
1	Penetration without perfusion; failure of contrast medium to move out of the area of occlusion
2	Partial perfusion; passage of contrast medium through obstruction but at a slow rate of clearance
3	Complete perfusion; prompt antegrade flow distal to the obstruction and adequate clearance of contrast medium

Table 2.2
TIMI Risk Score

Markers

- Age ≥65 yr
- ≥3 Coronary artery disease risk factors
- Known coronary artery disease with >50% stenosis
- ≥2 Anginal episodes within the past 24 h
- ST-segment deviation ≥0.5 mm on presenting electrocardiogram (ECG)
- Elevated cardiac markers

From: *Pocket Guide to Critical Care Pharmacotherapy*
By: J. Papadopoulos © Humana Press Inc., Totowa, NJ

- Aspirin in the past 7 d

Number of markers and 14-d risk of death, myocardial infarction, or urgent revascularization

- 0/1 – 4.7%
- 2 – 8.3%
- 3 – 13.2%
- 4 – 19.9%
- 5 – 26.2%
- 6/7 – 40.9%

JAMA 2000;284:835–842.

Notes:
With an increasing risk factor score, progressively greater benefit is seen with:

(a) Enoxaparin vs unfractionated heparin.
(b) Tirofiban vs placebo.
(c) Invasive strategy vs conservative strategy.

Table 2.3
Short-Term Risk of Death or Nonfatal Myocardial Infarction in Patients Presenting With Unstable Angina

Feature	High-risk (≥2 present)	Intermediate-risk (≥1 present)
History	• Increased tempo of signs/symptoms in preceding 48 h	• Prior to myocardial infarction, coronary artery bypass graft (CABG), peripheral artery disease, cerebrovascular accident, or aspirin use
Pain	• Pain at rest lasting >20 min	• Pain at rest lasting >20 min now resolved, with moderate or high likelihood of coronary artery disease • Rest angina lasting <20 min relieved with rest or sublingual nitroglycerin

(Continued)

Table 2.3 *(Continued)*

Feature	High-risk (≥2 present)	Intermediate-risk (≥1 present)
Clinical findings	• Pulmonary edema • New/worsening rales • New/worsening MR murmur • S_3 gallop • Hypotension • Tachycardia • Bradycardia • Age >75 yr	• Age >70 yr
Electrocardiogram	• ST-segment changes >0.05 mV	• T-wave inversions >0.2 mV • Pathological Q-waves
(ECG) findings	• New bundle-branch block • Sustained ventricular tachycardia	
Cardiac markers	• Troponin T or I > 0.1 ng/mL	• Troponin T or I > 0.01 but <0.1 ng/mL

J. Am. Coll. Cardiol. 2000;36:970–1062.

Note: low-risk omitted.

Table 2.4
Acute Pharmacological Management of Unstable Angina and Non-ST Elevation Myocardial Infarction

Antithrombotic pharmacotherapy
- Aspirin (if no evidence of allergy)
  - 162–325 mg chew and swallow immediately, followed by 75–162 mg enterally daily (indefinitely)
    - If history of aspirin-induced bleeding or bleeding risk factors present, use lower doses (i.e., 75–81 mg daily)
- Clopidogrel
  - In patients with an aspirin allergy or major aspirin gastrointestinal intolerance
    - 300 mg enterally in one dose, followed by 75 mg daily

- o In patients in whom an early noninvasive approach is planned (catheterization will be delayed [>24–36 h] or if coronary artery bypass graft [CABG] will not occur for >5 d following angiography)
  - ■ 300 mg enterally in one dose, followed by 75 mg daily for at least 1 mo and up to 9–12 mo in addition to aspirin pharmacotherapy
    - □ Do not use combination therapy in patients at high risk of bleeding or if the need for urgent CABG cannot be excluded
  - o If angiography will occur within 24 h initiate clopidogrel pharmacotherapy in the catheterization laboratory before percutaneous coronary intervention (PCI) or immediately after the procedure
- Glycoprotein IIb/IIIa inhibitors
  - o Administered, in addition to aspirin and heparin, to patients in whom catheterization and PCI are planned. May be administered just before PCI
  - o Either eptifibatide or tirofiban can be administered for initial early treatment in addition to aspirin (and/or clopidogrel) and low molecular weight heparin (LMWH) or heparin in *intermediate to high-risk patients* in whom an invasive management strategy is not planned (*see* Table 2.3 for risk assessment)
  - o Abciximab is not indicated in patients in whom PCI is not planned
- Unfractionated heparin
  - o In combination with antiplatelet pharmacotherapy
  - o Weight-based dosing to achieve an activated partial thromboplastin time (aPTT) between 50 and 70 s
    - ■ 60–70 units/kg IV bolus (4000 units maximum), followed by 12–15 units/kg/h continuous IV infusion (1000 units/h maximum)
  - o Nomogram for adjusting the heparin infusion

aPTT (s)	Rebolus	Stop infusion	Change infusion
<35	80 units/kg	–	↑ by 4 units/kg/h
35–49	40 units/kg	–	↑ by 2 units/kg/h
50–70	–	–	–
71–90	–	–	↓ by 2 units/kg/h
>90	–	1 h	↓ by 3 units/kg/h

- ■ If patient is obese, utilize an adjusted body weight for heparin dosing
  - □ Adjusted body weight = ideal body weight + 0.3 (actual body weight – ideal body weight)
- ■ Check aPTT every 6 h until stable then every 12–24 h
- ○ Use beyond 48 h is indicated in patients with refractory or recurrent angina or a large infarction
- • Low molecular weight heparins (adjust dose for renal dysfunction [i.e., creatinine clearance <30 mL/min])
  - ○ Enoxaparin may be preferred over unfractionated heparin in intermediate to high-risk patients (*see* Table 2.3 for risk assessment)
  - ○ Enoxaparin
    - ■ 1 mg/kg SQ every 12 h for 2–8 d
  - ○ Dalteparin
    - ■ 120 units/kg SQ every 12 h for 5–8 d
    - ■ Maximum dose = 10,000 units

Anti-ischemic pharmacotherapy
- • β-adrenergic blockers
  - ○ *Avoid early* if cocaine-induced acute coronary syndrome or evidence of cardiogenic shock or systemic hypoperfusion
  - ○ Intravenous agents
    - ■ Atenolol
      - □ 5 mg IV over 5 min. May repeat dose in 10 min
      - □ Step down to 50–100 mg enterally daily if tolerated
        - ♦ Adjust dose for renal dysfunction
    - ■ Metoprolol
      - □ 5mg for IV every 5 min in three doses
      - □ Step down to 50 mg enterally q6h × 48 h then 100 mg enterally bid if tolerated
    - ■ Propranolol
      - □ 1 mg slow intravenous push (IVP), repeated every 5 min. Not to exceed a total of 5 mg
      - □ An alternative dosing regimen may be 0.1 mg/kg in three divided doses every 2–3 min. Do not exceed a rate of 1 mg/min
  - ○ Contraindications

- Bradycardia (heart rate <60 bpm), systolic blood pressure <100 mmHg, severe left ventricular dysfunction with pulmonary edema, second- or third-degree heart block, PR interval >0.24 s, evidence of hypoperfusion, active asthma
    - Avoid β-adrenergic blockers with intrinsic sympathomimetic activity (e.g., acebutolol, pindolol)
- Nitroglycerin
    - Sublingual 0.4 mg tablets every 5 min × three doses on presentation. Initiate intravenous pharmacotherapy if chest pain persists
    - Start continuous IV infusion at 5–10 mcg/min and titrate using 5–10 mcg/min increments until symptoms resolve or systolic blood pressure (SBP) <90 mmHg or mean arterial pressure (MAP) falls by ≥30 mmHg from baseline. Usual maximum dose = 200 mcg/min
    - Avoid in patients with:
        - Right ventricular infarction
        - If presenting SBP is <90 mmHg or ≥30 mmHg below baseline MAP
        - Presence of profound bradycardia or tachycardia
        - Recent use (within 24 h of sildenafil or vardenafil or within 48 h of tadalafil) of a phosphodiesterase-5 inhibitor for erectile dysfunction (or pulmonary hypertension)
    - Use beyond 48 h is indicated in patients with persistent angina or pulmonary congestion
    - Dilates large coronary arteries and collateral vessels
    - Some intravenous preparations contain significant amounts of ethanol

Adjuvant pharmacotherapy
- Angiotensin converting enzyme inhibitors (ACE-I)—(oral therapy within 24 h after presentation)
    - Greatest benefit in patients with left ventricular dysfunction (ejection fraction [EF] <40%), anterior wall infarction, or pulmonary congestion. Use without these conditions is still warranted
    - Angiotensin receptor blockers if allergic or intolerant to ACE-I (data with valsartan and candesartan)

- ○ Start with low doses and increase as tolerated
- ○ Low doses of aspirin (i.e., 75–162 mg) may minimize any potential interaction with ACE-Is
- Statins (and National Cholesterol Education Program Adult Treatment Panel III diet)
  - ○ Low density lipoprotein (LDL) goal is patient specific
    - ▪ Very high-risk patients may benefit from target LDL goals <70 mg/dL
  - ○ Commence therapy within 24–96 h after admission
    - ▪ For example, atorvastatin 80 mg enterally daily
  - ○ If patient is on a statin before admission, continue therapy during admission to avoid rebound phenomenon
- Consider niacin or a fibrate for additional pharmacotherapy if high density lipoprotein (HDL) is <40 mg/dL
- Morphine
  - ○ 2–5 mg IV over 5 min every 5–30 min as needed
- Oxygen therapy
  - ○ Administer to patients with an SaO_2^- <90%
  - ○ Little justification for use beyond the first 2–6 h in the uncomplicated patient
- Sodium nitroprusside (dilates *only* large coronary arteries and *not* collateral vessels)
  - ○ May cause coronary steal. Avoid general utilization in patients with acute coronary syndromes. If therapy is indicated, use in combination with nitroglycerin, as this agent dilates large coronary arteries and collateral vessels

Chest 2004;126:513S–548S.
Circulation 2003;108(suppl III):III-28–III-37.
Circulation 2002;106:1893–1900.

Table 2.5

Acute Pharmacological Management of ST-Elevation Myocardial Infarction (Noninvasive or Conservative Strategy)

Fibrinolytic pharmacotherapy (in the absence of contraindications)

- Indicated for patients with ischemic symptoms of ≤12 h in duration and 12-lead electrocardiogram (ECG) evidence of:

- o ST-elevation >0.1 mV in at least two contiguous precordial leads or at least two adjacent limb leads
  - Some beneficial evidence exists to support administration times of up to 24 h after symptom onset in patients with continuous ischemic symptoms
- o New (or presumed new) left-bundle-branch block
- o A true posterior wall infarction
  - May manifest as tall R waves in the right precordial leads and ST-segment depression in leads $V_1 - V_4$
- Alteplase, reteplase, or tenecteplase preferred over strepto kinase in:
  - o Patients with symptom duration ≤6 h
  - o Anterior wall infarction (large area of injury)
- Administration within 30 min of arrival into the healthcare system recommended
- Exclude contraindications (*see* Table 2.7)

Agents for IV administration
- Alteplase (tPA)
  - o 15 mg IV bolus followed by 0.75 mg/kg continuous IV infusion (not to exceed 50 mg) over 30 min, followed by 0.5 mg/kg continuous IV infusion (not to exceed 35 mg) over 1 h
- Reteplase (rPA)
  - o 10 units IV push over 2 min followed 30 min later with another 10 units IV push over 2 min (administer a normal saline flush with each dose)
- Tenecteplase (TNKase)—single dose IV push over 5 s
  - o <60kg—30 mg
  - o 60–69.9 kg—35 mg
  - o 70–79.9 kg—40 mg
  - o 80–89.9 kg—45 mg
  - o ≥90 kg—50 mg
- Streptokinase
  - o 1.5 million units continuous IV infusion over 60 min using a ≥0.45 μm inline filter
  - o Monitor for any signs of an allergic reaction
  - o Antibodies remain for at least 3–6 mo after administration

Evidence of improvement
- Relief of presenting signs and symptoms
- Sustained hemodynamic and electrical stability
- A reduction of at least 50% of the ST-segment elevation on follow-up ECG obtained 60–90 min after fibrinolytic therapy

Adjuvant antithrombotic pharmacotherapy
- Aspirin (if no evidence of allergy)
  - 162–325 mg chew and swallow immediately, followed by 75–162 mg enterally daily (indefinitely)
    - If history of aspirin-induced bleeding or bleeding risk factors present, use lower doses (i.e., 81 mg daily)
- Clopidogrel
  - In patients with an aspirin allergy or major aspirin gastrointestinal intolerance
    - 300 mg enterally in one dose, followed by 75 mg daily
  - Combination clopidogrel 75 mg daily and aspirin 162 mg daily (up to 4 wk) in patients who did not receive percutaneous coronary intervention (PCI) has been shown to be effective in one clinical trial
    - Do not use combination therapy in patients at high-risk for bleeding or if the need for urgent coronary artery bypass graft (CABG) cannot be excluded
- Unfractionated heparin
  - As adjunct therapy to the use of alteplase, reteplase, and tenecteplase
    - 60 units/kg IV bolus (4000 units maximum), followed by 12 units/kg/h continuous IV infusion (1000 units/h maximum)
  - For patients receiving streptokinase
    - Recommended if patient is at high-risk of systemic thromboembolism (anterior wall infarction, heart failure, left ventricular thrombus, atrial fibrillation, previous embolism)
  - Weight-based dosing to achieve an activated partial thromboplastin time (aPTT) between 50 and 70 s
    - 60–70 units/kg IV bolus (4000 units maximum), followed by 12–15 units/kg/h continuous IV infusion (1000 units/h maximum)
  - Nomogram for adjusting the heparin infusion

aPTT (s)	Rebolus	Stop infusion	Change infusion
<35	80 units/kg	–	↑ by 4 units/kg/h
35–49	40 units/kg	–	↑ by 2 units/kg/h
50–70	–	–	–
71–90	–	–	↓ by 2 units/kg/h
>90	–	1 h	↓ by 3 units/kg/h

- ▪ If patient is obese, utilize an adjusted body weight for heparin dosing
  - □ Adjusted body weight = ideal body weight + 0.3 (actual body weight – ideal body weight)
- ▪ Check aPTT every 6 h until stable then every 12–24 h
- ▪ For patients receiving *concomitant* fibrinolytic pharmacotherapy, check an aPTT 3 h after heparin initiation
- ○ Use beyond 48 h is indicated in patients with refractory or recurrent angina or a large infarction
- • Warfarin
  - ○ In aspirin allergic or intolerant patients or as an alternative to clopidogrel with an indication for anticoagulation
    - ▪ Monotherapy to achieve an international normalized ratio (INR) between 2.5 and 3.5
    - ▪ Dose to achieve an INR between 2 and 3 if concomitant atrial fibrillation or atrial flutter
  - ○ In patients with a large anterior wall infarction and significant left ventricular dysfunction, visible intracardiac thrombus, akinetic segment, or a history of a thromboembolic event
    - ▪ Administered to achieve an INR of 2.5 (range 2–3) in combination with low-dose aspirin pharmacotherapy (≤100 mg daily [*Chest* guidelines] or 75–162 mg daily [*Circulation* guidelines]) for 3 mo postmyocardial infarction. Repeat echocardiogram before discontinuing warfarin pharmacotherapy

Anti-ischemic pharmacotherapy
- • β-adrenergic blockers
  - ○ *Avoid early* if cocaine-induced acute coronary syndrome or evidence of cardiogenic shock or systemic hypoperfusion
  - ○ Intravenous agents
    - ▪ Atenolol
      - □ 5 mg IV over 5 min. May repeat dose in 10 min
      - □ Step down to 50–100 mg enterally daily if tolerated

- ♦ Adjust dose for renal dysfunction
  - Metoprolol
    - □ 5 mg IV for every 5 min in three doses
    - □ Step down to 50 mg enterally q6h × 48 h then 100 mg enterally bid if tolerated
  - Propranolol
    - □ 1 mg slow intravenous push (IVP), repeated every 5 min. Not to exceed a total of 5 mg
    - □ An alternative dosing regimen may be 0.1 mg/kg in three divided doses every 2–3 min. Do not exceed a rate of 1 mg/min
  - ○ Contraindications
    - Bradycardia (heart rate <60 bpm), systolic blood pressure <100 mmHg, severe left ventricular dysfunction with pulmonary edema, second or third-degree heart block, PR interval >0.24s, evidence of hypoperfusion, active asthma
  - ○ Avoid β-adrenergic blockers with intrinsic sympathomimetic activity (e.g., acebutolol, pindolol)
- Nitroglycerin
  - ○ Sublingual 0.4 mg tablets every 5 min × three doses on presentation. Initiate intravenous pharmacotherapy if chest pain persists
  - ○ Start continuous IV infusion at 5–10 mcg/min and titrate using 5–10 mcg/min increments until symptoms resolve or systolic blood pressure (SBP) <90 mmHg or mean arterial pressure (MAP) falls by ≥30 mmHg from baseline. Usual maximum dose = 200 mcg/min
  - ○ Avoid in patients with:
    - Right ventricular infarction
    - If presenting systolic blood pressure (SBP) is <90 mmHg or ≥30 mmHg below baseline MAP
    - Presence of profound bradycardia or tachycardia
    - Recent use (within 24 h of sildenafil or vardenafil or within 48 h of tadalafil) of a phosphodiesterase-5 inhibitor for erectile dysfunction (or pulmonary hypertension)
  - ○ Use beyond 48 h is indicated in patients with persistent angina or pulmonary congestion
  - ○ Dilates large coronary arteries and collateral vessels
  - ○ Some intravenous preparations contain significant amounts of ethanol

Adjuvant pharmacotherapy
- Angiotensin converting enzyme inhibitors (ACE-I)—(oral therapy within 24 h after presentation)
  ○ Greatest benefit in patients with left ventricular dysfunction (ejection fraction <40%), anterior wall infarction, or pulmonary congestion. Use without these conditions is still warranted
    ▪ Use indefinitely in patients with left ventricular dysfunction
    ▪ Use for 4–6 wk in patients without left ventricular dysfunction unless another indication exists
  ○ Angiotensin receptor blockers (ARBs) if allergic or intolerant to ACE-I (data with valsartan and candesartan)
  ○ Start with low doses and increase as tolerated
  ○ Low doses of aspirin (i.e., 75–162 mg) may minimize any potential interaction with ACE-Is
- Calcium channel blockers (verapamil or diltiazem only)
  ○ May be utilized in situations where β-adrenergic blockers are ineffective or contraindicated
  ○ Do not use a calcium channel blocker in the setting of chronic heart failure, 2° or 3° atrioventricular block, or left ventricular dysfunction
- Aldosterone receptor blockade
  ○ Spironolactone 25 mg enterally daily or eplerenone 25 mg enterally daily
    ▪ May increase spironolactone or eplerenone to 50 mg daily within 4 wk
  ○ Indicated in patients on ACE-I or ARB pharmacotherapy with a left ventricular ejection fraction ≤40% and either symptomatic heart failure or diabetes mellitus
    ▪ Contraindications include serum potassium >5.5 mEq/L at initiation or a creatinine clearance ≤30 mL/min. Eplerenone is a CYP3A4 substrate
- Statins (and National Cholesterol Education Program Adult Treatment Panel III diet)
  ○ Low density lipoprotein (LDL) goal is patient-specific

- ▪ Very high-risk patients may benefit from target LDL goals <70 mg/dL
  - ○ Commence therapy within 24–96 h after admission
    - ▪ For example, atorvastatin 80 mg enterally daily
  - ○ If patient is on a statin before admission, continue therapy during admission to avoid rebound phenomenon
- Consider niacin or a fibrate for additional pharmacotherapy if high density lipoprotein (HDL) is <40 mg/dL
- Morphine
  - ○ 2–5 mg IV over 5 min every 5–30 min as needed
- Oxygen therapy
  - ○ Administer to patients with an SaO_2^- <90%
  - ○ Little justification for use beyond the first 2–6 h in the uncomplicated patient
- Sodium nitroprusside (dilates *only* large coronary arteries and *not* collateral vessels)
  - ○ May cause coronary steal. Avoid general utilization in patients with acute coronary syndromes. If therapy is indicated, use in combination with nitroglycerin, as this agent dilates large coronary arteries and collateral vessels
- Insulin infusions (controversial)
  - ○ Patient should have a continuous source of dextrose
  - ○ In patients with hyperglycemia with or without pre-existing diabetes
  - ○ During the first 24–48 h (especially in patients with a complicated course)
  - ○ Maintain blood glucose between 80 and 140 mg/dL
    - ▪ Optimum range not delineated
    - ▪ Strict avoidance of hypoglycemia is advocated
- Docusate sodium 100 mg enterally tid to prevent straining
- Anxiolytic medications as needed

Chest 2004;126:549S–575S.
Circulation 2004;110:E82–E292.
Lancet 2005;366:1607–1621.

Table 2.6
Considerations in Patients With Right
Ventricular Infarctions

- Obtain right precordial leads in any patient with an inferior wall myocardial infarction
- Patients have an exaggerated preload dependence. Blood pressure may decrease in response to diuretics, nitroglycerin, morphine, and/or positive end expiratory pressure (PEEP) or continuous positive air pressure (CPAP)
  - ○ Judicious use of fluids to maintain normal jugular venous pressure
    - ■ Excess fluid may be harmful (i.e., shift intraventricular septum into left ventricle, increase right ventricular oxygen demand)
  - ○ Careful use of nitroglycerin, loop diuretics, and morphine
    - ■ All can result in venous dilation with a resultant decrease in preload
- Restore atrioventricular synchrony if possible
- Reduce right-ventricular afterload
- Avoid hypoxemia, acidosis, and lung hyperinflation

Table 2.7
Contraindications to Fibrinolytic Therapy in Patients
With ST-Elevation Myocardial Infarction

Absolute	*Relative*
• Active internal bleeding (except menses)	• History of chronic, severe, uncontrolled hypertension
• Previous hemorrhagic stroke	• Uncontrolled hypertension on presentation (>180/110 mmHg)
• Atherothrombotic or cardioembolic cerebrovascular accident within 3 mo	
• Known intracranial neoplasm (primary or metastatic), aneurysm, arteriovenous malformation	• Current use of anticoagulants in therapeutics doses
	• Known bleeding diathesis
	• Recent internal bleeding (within 2–4 wk)

(Continued)

Table 2.7 *(Continued)*

Absolute	Relative
• Suspected aortic dissection • Significant closed-head injury or facial trauma within 3 mo	• Recent major surgery (within 3 wk) • Recent trauma (within 2–4 wk) • Recent prolonged cardiopulmonary resuscitation (>10 min) with evidence of thoracic trauma • Lumbar puncture within 7 d • Noncompressible vascular punctures • Active peptic ulcer disease • Pregnancy • For streptokinase/anistreplase—previous exposure (>5 d ago) or documented allergy

Table 2.8
Management of Acute Decompensated Heart Failure

Pulmonary edema only
- Furosemide 0.5–1 mg/kg IV push
- Morphine 2–4 mg IV
- Nitroglycerin sublingual/IV if hemodynamically stable
- Oxygen/positive end expiratory pressure (PEEP)/intubation as needed

Hypoperfusion state only
- Crystalloid/colloid to achieve a pulmonary capillary wedge pressure (PCWP) between 15 and 18 mmHg
  - If cardiac index (CI) >2.2 L/min/m^2 and patient improves clinically → observe
- If PCWP between 15 and 18 mmHg and symptomatic
  - If adequate mean arterial pressure (MAP)

- Dobutamine—2.5–10 mcg/kg/min continuous IV infusion up to 20 mcg/kg/min
- Milrinone—0.2–0.75 mcg/kg/min continuous IV infusion
  □ Loading dose of 50 mcg/kg over 10 min may be utilized
    ◆ Avoid or administer 50% if tenuous hemodynamics
  □ Use lower doses in patients with renal dysfunction (i.e., 0.2 mcg/kg/min)
  □ Limited experience with dobutamine and milrinone coadministration
- Add nitroprusside or nesiritide if CI <2.2 L/min/m^2 and clinical end point not achieved despite therapeutic dobutamine +/– milrinone
  □ Nitroprusside—0.25–0.5 mcg/kg/min continuous IV infusion; increase in increments of 0.25–0.5 mcg/kg/min until desired hemodynamic effect. Usual doses up to 2–3 mcg/kg/min.
    High-alert medication—read package insert before use
  □ Nesiritide—2 mcg/kg IV bolus followed by a continuous IV infusion of 0.01 mcg/kg/min. Doses above the initial infusion rate should be limited to carefully selected patients. High-alert medication—read package insert before use
- If inadequate MAP
  ○ Dopamine—2.5–20 mcg/kg/min continuous IV infusion. May require doses ≥10 mcg/kg/min for adequate BP response
  ○ Norepinephrine—start at 4 mcg/min and titrate to desired effect

Pulmonary congestion and hypoperfusion
- If adequate MAP
  ○ Goal PCWP between 15 and 18 mmHg
  ○ Furosemide 0.5–1 mg/kg IV push

- ■ +/– morphine 2–4 mg IV
- ■ +/– nitroglycerin IV
  - □ Start continuous IV infusion at 5–10 mcg/min and titrate using 5–10 mcg/min increments until symptoms resolve or SBP <90 mmHg or MAP falls by ≥30 mmHg from baseline. Usual maximum dose = 200 mcg/min
  - ○ Dobutamine—2.5–10 mcg/kg/min continuous IV infusion up to 20 mcg/kg/min
  - ○ Milrinone—0.2–0.75 mcg/kg/min continuous IV infusion
    - ■ Loading dose of 50 mcg/kg over 10 min may be utilized
      - □ Avoid or administer 50% if tenuous hemodynamics
    - ■ Use lower doses in patients with renal dysfunction (i.e., 0.2 mcg/kg/min)
    - ■ Limited experience with dobutamine and milrinone coadministration
- • If inadequate MAP
  - ○ Goal PCWP between 15 and 18 mmHg
  - ○ Furosemide 0.5–1 mg/kg IV
    - ■ +/– morphine 2–4 mg IV
  - ○ Dopamine—2.5–20 mcg/kg/min continuous IV infusion. May require doses ≥10 mcg/kg/min for adequate BP response
  - ○ Norepinephrine — start at 4 mcg/min and titrate to desired effect

Notes:

(a) CI and PCWP values for patients with pulmonary artery catheterization.

(b) Continuous positive air pressure (CPAP) may provide preload and afterload reduction and improve oxygenation and work of breathing in patients with acute pulmonary edema.

(c) Balloon pump may be considered in patients with or without acute coronary syndrome or in patients with cardiogenic shock with adequate filling pressures.

Table 2.9
Vaughan Williams Classification of Antiarrhythmics

Type	Drug	Automaticity	Conduction velocity	Refractory period	Blockade
Ia[a]	Quinidine Procainamide[b] Disopyramide	→	→	↑	Sodium (intermediate)
Ib	Lidocaine Mexiletine Tocainide	→	0/↓	→	Sodium (fast on–off)
Ic	Flecainide Propafenone[c] Moricizine	→	↓↓	0	Sodium (slow on–off)
II	β-adrenergic blockers[d]	→	→	↑	β-adrenergic receptors

(Continued)

Table 2.9 (Continued)

Type	Drug	Automaticity	Conduction velocity	Refractory period	Blockade
III[e]	Amiodarone[f] Sotalol[c] Ibutelide Dofelitide	0	0	↑↑	Potassium
IV	Verapamil Diltiazem	↓	↓	↑	Calcium

[a]Class I antiarrhythmics display different binding affinity for the sodium channel (C > A > B). They possess rate-dependence properties (i.e., sodium channel blockade is greatest at fast heart rates). Additionally, this class may increase defibrillation threshold (i.e., greater energy may be required for successful cardioversion).

[b]The N-acetyl procainamide (NAPA) metabolite blocks rapid potassium channels.

[c]Has β-blocking properties.

[d]Propranolol (at high doses) has been noted to have quinidine-like activity.

[e]This class may decrease defibrillation threshold (i.e., less energy may be required for successful cardioversion).

[f]Has activity of all four Vaughan Williams classifications.

39

Table 2.10
Antithrombotic Pharmacotherapy for Patients
With Various Diseases

Atrial fibrillation (paroxysmal, persistent, or chronic)
- *Risk factors* for embolic cerebrovascular accidents include previous ischemic stroke, transient ischemic attacks (TIA), systemic embolism, age >75 yr, moderately or severely impaired left ventricular systolic function, hypertension, diabetes mellitus
  - <65 yr of age and no risk factors—aspirin 325 mg daily
  - <65 yr of age and one or more risk factors—warfarin administered to achieve an international normalized ratio (INR) of 2.5 (range 2–3)
  - 65–75 yr of age and no risk factors—warfarin administered to achieve an INR of 2.5 (range 2–3) or aspirin 325 mg daily
  - 65–75 yr of age and one or more risk factors—warfarin administered to achieve an INR of 2.5 (range 2–3)
  - >75 yr of age—warfarin administered to achieve an INR of 2.5 (range 2–3)
- Some clinicians advocate the use of a $CHADS_2$ score to assess thromboembolic risk
  - Congestive heart failure (1 point)
  - Hypertension (1 point)
  - Age ≥75 yr (1 point)
  - Diabetes mellitus (1 point)
  - Secondary (previous) TIA, CVA, or systemic embolic event prevention (2 points)
  - Low-risk score = 0, intermediate risk score = 1–2, high-risk score ≥3
- Atrial fibrillation and mitral stenosis
  - Warfarin administered to achieve an INR of 2.5 (range 2–3)
- Elective cardioversion (≥48 h)
  - Warfarin administered to achieve an INR of 2.5 (range 2–3) for 3 wk before elective cardioversion and for at least 4 wk after successful cardioversion

- ○ If < 48 h in duration, can perform with intravenous unfractionated heparin or full dose low molecular weight heparin (LMWH) at presentation
- Transesophageal (TEE)-guided elective cardioversion
  - ○ Intravenous unfractionated heparin (goal activated partial thromboplastin time [aPTT] = 60 s [range 50–70 s]) or at least 5 d of warfarin administered to achieve an INR of 2.5 (range 2–3)
    - If no thrombus is observed and cardioversion is successful, continue warfarin pharmacotherapy for 4 wk
    - If thrombus is observed, postpone cardioversion and continue anticoagulation indefinitely
- Emergency cardioversion
  - ○ Intravenous unfractionated heparin (goal activated partial thromboplastin time [aPTT] = 60 s [range 50–70 s]) started as soon as possible followed by 4 wk of warfarin administered to achieve an INR of 2.5 (range 2–3)
- Atrial flutter cardioversion
  - ○ Same as atrial fibrillation

Rheumatic mitral valve disease
- *And* history of atrial fibrillation or previous systemic embolism
  - ○ Warfarin administered to achieve an INR of 2.5 (range 2–3). Do not combine with an antiplatelet agent
  - ○ If patient experiences a systemic embolism while receiving warfarin and has a therapeutic INR, add aspirin 75–100 mg/d. For patients unable to take aspirin, then add dipyridamole 400 mg/d or clopidogel 75 mg/d. Immediate release dipyridamole needs an acidic gastric pH (<4) for adequate absorption
- Normal sinus rhythm and a left atrial diameter >5.5 cm
  - ○ Warfarin administered to achieve an INR of 2.5 (range 2–3)
- Normal sinus rhythm and a left atrial diameter <5.5 cm
  - ○ No antithrombotic therapy recommended
- Undergoing mitral valvuloplasty
  - ○ Warfarin administered to achieve an INR of 2.5 (range 2–3) for 3 wk before procedure and for at least 4 wk after procedure

Prosthetic heart valves

- All patients with a mechanical prosthetic heart valve should receive concomitant unfractionated heparin *or* a low molecular weight heparin in combination with warfarin pharmacotherapy until the INR is therapeutic and stable for *two* consecutive days
- A St. Jude Medical bileaflet mechanical valve in the aortic position
  ○ Warfarin is administered to achieve an INR of 2.5 (range 2–3)
- Tilting disk valve and bileaflet mechanical valve in the mitral position
  ○ Warfarin is administered to achieve an INR of 3 (range 2.5–3.5)
- A CarboMetrics bileaflet valve or Medtronic Hall tilting disk mechanical valve in the aortic position, with normal left atrial size and normal sinus rhythm
  ○ Warfarin is administered to achieve an INR of 2.5 (range 2–3)
- Bileaflet mechanical valve *and* either atrial fibrillation, myocardial infarction, left atrial enlargement, endocardial damage, or low ejection fraction
  ○ Warfarin is administered to achieve an INR of 3 (range 2.5–3.5) in *combination* with aspirin 75–100 mg/d
- Caged ball or caged disk valves
  ○ Warfarin is administered to achieve an INR of 3 (range 2.5–3.5) in *combination* with aspirin 75–100 mg/d
- If a patient with a mechanical prosthetic heart valve suffer a systemic embolic event despite having a therapeutic INR
  ○ Add aspirin 75–100 mg/d and increase the level of anti-coagulation to achieve an INR of 3 (range 2.5–3.5)
- Bioprosthetic mitral valve
  ○ Warfarin is administered for 3 mo postoperatively to achieve an INR of 2.5 (range 2–3), then aspirin 75–100 mg/d
- Bioprosthetic aortic valve
  ○ Warfarin is administered for 3 mo postoperatively to achieve an INR of 2.5 (range 2–3) or aspirin 75–100 mg/d. Long-term therapy with aspirin 75–100 mg/d
- Bioprosthetic valve and atrial fibrillation
  ○ Warfarin is administered to achieve an INR of 2.5 (range 2–3)

Chest 2004;126:429S–482S.

Table 2.11
Causes and Management of Acquired Torsades de Pointes

Factors that may exacerbate/precipitate
- Congenital
  - Jervell–Lange–Nielsen (autosomal dominant with congenital deafness)
  - Romano-Ward (autosomal dominant without deafness)
- Severe bradycardia (<50 bpm), sinus node dysfunction, A-V block
- Cardiomyopathy, myocarditis, myocardial ischemia/ infarction
- Hypokalemia, hypomagnesemia, hypocalcemia
- Starvation, anorexia nervosa, and liquid protein diets
- Hypothyroidism, severe hypothermia
- Female sex
- Ion-channel polymorphisms

Medications (extensive list may be found at www.torsades.org)
- Antiarrhythmic agents
  - Quinidine, procainamide, disopyramide, sotalol, ibutilide, dofetilide, bepridil, and amiodarone (less common)
- Anti-infectives
  - Clarithromycin, erythromycin, telithromycin, fluoro-quinolones, pentamidine, amantadine, foscarnet, and voriconazole
- Antipsychotics
  - Chlorpromazine, thioridazine, mesoridazine, quetiapine, ziprasidone, haloperidol, and risperidone
- Antidepressants
  - Amitriptyline, desipramine, doxepin, imipramine, and venlafaxine
- Others
  - Tamoxifen, droperidol, cisapride, tizanidine, probucol, quinine, methadone, levomethadyl, and ranolazine
- Review medication profile for drug–drug interactions (extensive lists may be found at www.drug-interactions.com)

Management
- Discontinue offending drug(s)
- Unsynchronized electric defibrillation if hemodynamically unstable
- Correct any electrolyte disorders (e.g., hypokalemia, hypomagnesemia)
- Magnesium IV (suppresses early after-depolarizations)
  - 1–2 g IV in 50–100 mL D5W over 2–5 min. May repeat dose in 15 min
  - Followed with 0.5–1 g/h continuous IV infusion (titrate dose to control torsades de pointes)
- Temporary transvenous overdrive pacing (100 bpm)
- Pharmacological pacing
  - Isoproterenol 2–10 mcg/min continuous IV infusion (lower dose if patient has a history of coronary artery disease)
    - Titrate to increase heart rate (about 100 bpm) until torsades de pointes is suppressed
  - Epinephrine 2–10 mcg/min continuous IV infusion
    - Titrate to increase heart rate (about 100 bpm) until torsades de pointes is suppressed
- Lidocaine (less effective than above interventions)
- Sodium bicarbonate may be useful if torsades de pointes is because of quinidine

---

Table 2.12
Hypertensive Crises

Hypertensive emergency (no absolute blood pressure range)
- Sudden increase in systolic and diastolic blood pressure associated with end-organ damage. Organ dysfunction is uncommon with a diastolic blood pressure ≤120 mmHg. The absolute level may not be as important as the rate of increase. Lower blood pressure threshold for treatment in pregnant patients (i.e., ≥160–170/105–110 mmHg or mean arterial pressure >110 mmHg)

Hypertensive urgency
- Severely elevated blood pressure without acute end-organ damage

End-organ damage
- Heart
  - Acute aortic dissection, acute pulmonary edema, left ventricular failure, angina, and acute coronary syndrome
- Brain
  - Intracerebral hemorrhage (ICH), subarachnoid hemorrhage (SAH), and hypertensive encephalopathy
- Acute renal failure, visual deficits, microangiopathic hemolytic anemia, and pre-eclampsia/eclampsia

Diagnosis
- *Must* differentiate between hypertensive emergency and urgency
- History (previous crises, previous medications, recreational drug use), physical examination (mandatory fundoscopic examination, blood pressure on all limbs), urinalysis, and electrolytes, blood urea nitrogen, creatinine, peripheral blood smear, complete blood count, electrocardiogram (ECG), chest X-ray, and head CT
- Identify etiology if possible

Goals of blood pressure reduction
- Initial goal is *not* to achieve a normal BP (except in acute aortic dissection)
- Reduce mean arterial pressure (MAP) by 20–25% or to a diastolic blood pressure of 110 mmHg in hypertensive emergencies
- Reduce blood pressure gradually over 24–48 h in hypertensive urgencies

Hypertensive emergency	*Target/time to achieve goal*
- Acute aortic dissection	- SBP 100–120 mmHg and heart rate at 60 beats/min within 5–10 min
- Acute pulmonary edema	- MAP reduction within 15–30 min
- Hypertensive encephalopathy	- MAP reduction within 2–3 h

- Intracerebral hemorrhage
- BP 160/90 mmHg or MAP of 110 mmHg if there is no evidence or suspicion of elevated intracranial pressure. Time to achieve not well delineated (possibly within 3 h).
- Subarachnoid hemrrhage
- SBP between 140–160 mmHg within 3–6 h (no consensus)
- Catecholamine crisis
- MAP reduction within 2–6 h

Management of hypertensive emergencies (intravenous agents)
- Left ventricular failure and pulmonary edema
  ○ Drugs of choice—nitroprusside, nitroglycerin, fenoldopam, enalaprilat, loop diuretics, and nesiritide
  ○ Avoid—β-adrenergic blockers, nondihydropyridine calcium channel blockers, and hydralazine
- Acute coronary syndromes
  ○ Drugs of choice—nitroglycerin, β-adrenergic blockers, enalaprilat, nicardipine (may be added), and fenoldopam (may be added)
  ○ Cautious—nitroprusside (coronary steal phenomenon)
  ○ Avoid—hydralazine, minoxidil, diazoxide, and calcium channel blockers in Q-wave myocardial infarction
- Acute aortic dissection
  ○ Drugs of choice—esmolol + nitroprusside, esmolol + nicardipine, labetolol, and trimethophan
  ○ Avoid—hydralazine, minoxidil, and diazoxide
- Catecholamine crises
  ○ Drugs of choice—nitroprusside, phentolamine, nicardipine, and benzodiazepines in alcohol withdrawal or cocaine intoxications
  ○ Avoid—monotherapy with β-adrenergic blockers (including labetolol)
- Hypertensive encephalopathy, ICH, and SAH

- ○ Drugs of choice—labetolol, nimodipine (in SAH), fenoldopam, and nicardipine
  - ○ Avoid—nitroprusside, nitroglycerin, clonidine, methyldopa, propranolol, diazoxide, hydralazine, and minoxidil
- Acute renal failure/microangiopathic hemolytic anemia
  - ○ Drugs of choice—nicardipine, fenoldopam
  - ○ Avoid—nitroprusside, angiotensin converting enzyme inhibitors ACE-Is (except in sclerodermic renal crisis)
- Pre-eclampsia/eclampsia
  - ○ Drugs of choice—hydralazine, labetolol, and nicardipine
    - Hydralazine has a long history of safety in pregnancy; however, blood pressure lowering is unpredictable in timing and potency with a given intravenous dose (personal opinion)
  - ○ Avoid—nitroprusside, angiotensin converting enzyme inhibitors [ACE-Is], angiotensin receptor blockers [ARBs], and loop diuretics

Management of hypertensive urgencies (oral agents)
- Clonidine—0.2 mg enterally in one dose, then 0.1 mg q1h as needed to a total dose of 0.6 mg
- Captopril—25 mg enterally in one dose, then 12.5–25 mg as needed
- Labetolol—200–300 mg enterally every 2–3 h

Chest 2000;118:214–227.
Stroke 2007;38:2001–2023.

Table 2.13
Management of Catecholamine Extravasation

- Stop catecholamine infusion
- *Infiltrate* involved area with phentolamine 5 mg (in 10 mL normal saline)
  - ○ Use multiple small injections with a 27- or 30-gauge needle. Do not inject a volume that will result in skin swelling
- Repeat 5 mg if no evidence of resolution within 30 min

Table 2.14
Prevention of Venous Thromboembolism
in the Intensive Care Unit Patient

Review risk factors for thromboembolism
- Age >40 yr, previous venous thromboembolism, chronic heart failure, acute respiratory failure, recent major surgery (within 2 wk), confined air/ground travel (>6 h duration within 1 wk of admission), inflammatory bowel disease, myocardial infarction, nephrotic syndrome, and ischemic stroke
- Hypercoagulable states
  - Malignancy, sepsis, antiphospholipid antibody syndrome, dysfibrinogenemia, myeloproliferative disorders, hyperhomocysteinemia, and pregnancy/postpartum
  - Antithrombin, protein C, and protein S deficiencies
  - Factor V Leiden mutation, prothrombin 20210A gene mutation, and plasminogen activator inhibitor (PAI-1) excess
  - Heparin-induced thrombocytopenia
- Pharmacotherapy
  - Estrogen, megestrol, tamoxifen, and raloxifene, anesthesia use >40 min
- Vascular injury
  - Trauma, knee or hip surgery, and central venous access or in-dwelling femoral venous catheter
- Venous stasis
  - Immobility (including bedrest ≥3 d), paralysis, obesity, varicose veins, and hyperviscocity syndromes

Risk stratification
- Patients should be classified as low-, moderate-, or at high-risk depending on their medical condition and presence of risk factors

Prophylaxis
- Discontinue estrogen-containing products and megestrol based on clinical judgement
- Low-risk or if there is a contraindication to pharmacotherapy
  - Early ambulation *or* graduated compression stockings and/or intermittent pneumatic compression devices (IPC)
- Moderate-risk
  - Heparin 5000 units SQ q12h (*see* comment below)

- High-risk
  - IPC + heparin 5000 units SQ *q8h or* a low molecular weight heparin

Duration of prophylaxis
- Based on patient's medical condition and the presence or resolution of risk factors

---

Chest 2004;126:338S–400S.
Chest 2003;124:357S–363S.
Lancet 2002;359:849–850.

Notes:
(a) Prophylaxis is not indicated if the patient has therapeutic pharmacological anticoagulation.
(b) Pharmacotherapy should *not* be utilized if contraindications are present.
(c) Patients who weigh ≥70 kg should generally receive heparin 5000 units SQ q8h if moderate- or at high-risk.
(d) Patients on vasopressors may require higher doses or a different mode of drug administration.
(e) In patients with a creatinine clearance <30 mL/min, unfractionated heparin may be preferred. If a low molecular weight heparin is utilized, may need to adjust dose and monitor periodic antifactor-Xa levels to avoid drug accumulation.

Table 2.15
Management of Deep-Vein Thrombosis and Pulmonary Embolism

Deep-vein thrombosis
- Elevate and rest an acutely swollen leg
  - Routine bed rest should not be recommended as part of the standard of care
- Heparin
  - 80 units/kg IV bolus followed by 15–18 units/kg/h continuous IV infusion based on activated partial thromboplastin time (aPTT)
  - Nomogram for adjusting the heparin infusion

aPTT (s)	Rebolus	Stop infusion	Change infusion
<35	80 units/kg	–	↑ by 4 units/kg/h
35–49	40 units/kg	–	↑ by 2 units/kg/h

50–70	–	–	–
71–90	–	–	↓ by 2 units/kg/h
>90	–	1 h	↓ by 3 units/kg/h

- If patient is obese, utilize an adjusted body weight for heparin dosing
  - Adjusted body weight = ideal body weight + 0.3 (actual body weight – ideal body weight)
- Obtain aPTT every 6 h until stable, then every 12–24 h
- Obtain antifactor Xa levels to guide therapy in patients who require large doses of heparin (i.e., >25 units/kg/h)
- Low molecular weight heparins *(adjust doses for renal dysfunction)*
  - Dalteparin
    - 100 units/kg SQ q12h (maximum initial dose = 10,000 units)
  - Enoxaparin
    - 1 mg/kg SQ q12h (maximum initial dose = 180 mg)
  - Tinzaparin
    - 175 units/kg SQ q24h (maximum initial dose = 18,000 units/d)
- Fibrinolytic therapy
  - Systemic or local therapy reserved for patients who have limb-threatening thrombosis (phlegmasia cerulean dolens) despite appropriate heparin therapy
  - Consider venous thrombectomy if contraindications to fibrinolytic therapy exist
- Inferior vena cava filter
  - May be useful in patients with:
    - Contraindications to anticoagulation (e.g., serious bleeding risk, coagulopathic, thrombocytopenic, metastatic brain cancer, and fall risk)
    - Failure of anticoagulation
    - Low cardiopulmonary reserve (i.e., right-ventricular hypokinesis on echocardiogram) where an initial or repeat pulmonary embolism would be catastrophic
    - Large free-floating clot loosely attached to the inferior vena cava wall

Pulmonary embolism (PE)
- Not in shock, right ventricular dysfunction absent
  - Manage as deep vein thrombosis (DVT) protocol
- Not in shock and right ventricular dysfunction present
  - Manage as DVT protocol
  - Consider fibrinolysis in patients with persistent or worsening respiratory failure and/or evidence of hypoperfusion with a low risk of bleeding
- In shock (obstructive)
  - Volume expansion with a crystalloid or colloid
    - Excess fluid administration may increase right-ventricular (RV) wall stress, RV ischemia, tricuspid regurgitation, and cause a septal shift that may impair left-ventricular (LV) compliance and filling. Administer with caution in patients with documented severe RV dysfunction or when measured pressures are high
  - Vasopressor
    - Norepinephrine (preferred agent)
  - Fibrinolytic
    - Alteplase 100 mg IV over 2 h
    - Alteplase 0.6 mg/kg (maximum of 50 mg) over 2–15 min may be utilized if the patient is hemodynamically unstable or in cardiac arrest
    - Administer heparin without a loading dose when aPTT ≤2 × control after fibrinolysis
  - Embolectomy
    - Surgical embolectomy may be an alternative to IV thrombolysis in patients with decompensated shock (no prospective clinical trials)
    - Catheter-based embolectomy—limited experience in shock (not appropriate for patients with decompensated shock [personal opinion])

Long-term management
- Convert to warfarin pharmacotherapy
  - Start at the time of DVT/PE diagnosis when feasible

- ○ Target international normalized ratio (INR) 2.5 (range 2.0–3.0)
- ○ INR must be stable and therapeutic for *two* consecutive days before heparin or low molecular weight heparin is discontinued
- Patients with cancer who develop a venous thromboembolism may benefit from long-term therapy with a low molecular weight heparin (at least the first 3–6 mo of pharmacotherapy) instead of oral warfarin
  - ○ Data with:
    - Dalteparin 200 units/kg SQ daily for 1 mo, followed by 150 units/kg SQ daily thereafter
    - Tinzaparin 175 units/kg SQ daily
- Duration of DVT/PE pharmacotherapy
  - ○ First episode secondary to transient (reversible) risk factor(s)—3 mo
  - ○ First episode of an idiopathic event—6–12 mo (consider indefinite anticoagulation)
  - ○ First episode and presence of a malignancy—indefinite or until cancer resolves
  - ○ First episode with thrombophilia—12 mo (consider indefinite anticoagulation)
  - ○ Recurrent episode—indefinite
  - ○ Chronic thromboembolic pulmonary hypertension—indefinite

Chest 2004;126:401S–428S.
Circulation 2004;110(suppl):I3–I18.
NEJM 2004;351:268–277.
Chest 2002;121:877–905.

Table 2.16

Management of Elevated International Normalized Ratio (INR) in Patients Receiving Warfarin Pharmacotherapy

INR <5.0; no significant signs of bleeding	• Lower or omit dose • Monitor more frequently • Resume lower dose when INR in therapeutic range
INR ≥5.0 but <9.0; no	• Omit next one or two dose(s)

significant signs of bleeding	• Monitor more frequently • Resume lower dose when INR in therapeutic range
	Alternatively • Omit dose • Administer vitamin K_1 (1–2.5 mg enterally), especially if at increased risk of bleeding • If more rapid reversal is indicated, administer vitamin K_1 (2–4 mg enterally) • If the INR is still high after 24 h, additional vitamin K_1 (1–2 mg enterally) may be administered

INR ≥9.0; no significant signs of bleeding	• Hold warfarin pharmacotherapy
	• Administer vitamin K_1 (5–10 mg enterally)
	  ○ INR will be reduced in 24 h
	  ○ Administer more vitamin K_1 as needed
	• Monitor more frequently
	• Resume lower dose when INR in therapeutic range

Serious bleeding at any INR	• Hold warfarin pharmacotherapy • Administer vitamin K_1 (10 mg IV over 30 min) ○ May be repeated in 12 h • Supplement with fresh frozen plasma (15–20 mL/kg) or prothrombin complex concentrate • Recombinant factor VIIa may be considered as an alternative to prothrombin complex concentrate

| Life-threatening bleeding | • Hold warfarin pharmacotherapy
• Administer vitamin K_1 (10 mg IV over 30 min)
  ○ May be repeated in 12 h
• Supplement with fresh frozen plasma (15–20 mL/kg) or prothrombin complex concentrate
• Recombinant factor VIIa may be considered as an alternative to prothrombin complex concentrate |

Chest 2004;126:204S–233S.

Notes:

(a) When bleeding is not evident, goal of INR with intervention is to achieve a therapeutic INR (e.g., between 2 and 3; *not* 1).

(b) In patients with mild-to-moderate elevations in INR and no evidence of *major* bleeding, vitamin K_1 should be administered enterally rather than subcutaneously. Subcutaneous absorption may be erratic. The injectable preparation can be administered enterally when a patient needs <5 mg dose.

(c) Investigate the reason for the elevated INR (e.g., compliance, drug–drug interactions, drug–herbal interactions, drug–nutrient interactions, dietary changes).

(d) In patients who have bled and warfarin pharmacotherapy is reinitiated, consider lowering the intensity of anticoagulation.

(e) If systemic anticoagulation is warranted after high dose of vitamin K_1 (i.e., 10 mg), then the use of unfractionated heparin or a low molecular weight heparin (LMWH) may be required until the effects of vitamin K_1 are reversed and the patient becomes responsive to warfarin pharmacotherapy.

(f) The intravenous product, vitamin K, is an aqueous colloidal solution that contains a polyoxyethylated castor oil diluent. An anaphylactoid reaction can occur if the intravenous rate exceeds 1 mg/min.

Cerebrovascular

Table 3.1

General Supportive Care for Patients With an Acute Cerebrovascular Accident

- Airway support and ventilatory assistance in patients with a depressed level of consciousness or airway compromise
- Supplemental oxygen in hypoxic patients
- Antipyretics and cooling devices for the management of fever
- Antihypertensive agents should be avoided unless the systolic blood pressure is >220 mmHg or the diastolic blood pressure is >120 mmHg (*see* Table 3.2 for management)
  - ○ Patients who are otherwise eligible (except blood pressure) for alteplase, should have their blood pressure lowered cautiously to a systolic ≤185 mmHg and a diastolic ≤110 mmHg
- Treat hypotension with normal saline
- Avoid/treat hypoglycemia
- Control hyperglycemia
  - ○ Target blood glucose levels 80–140 mg/dL
    - ■ Optimal range not well delineated
    - ■ Frequent monitoring of blood glucose levels and adjustments of insulin are required to avoid hypoglycemia

Stroke 2007;38:1655–1711.
Chest 2004;126:483S–512S.
Stroke 2003;34:1056–1083.
NEJM 1995;333:1581–1587.
Guidelines 2000 for Cardiopulmonary Resuscitation and Emergency Cardiovascular Care. *Circulation* 2000;102(8):I86–I165.

From: *Pocket Guide to Critical Care Pharmacotherapy*
By: J. Papadopoulos © Humana Press Inc., Totowa, NJ

Table 3.2
Blood Pressure Management in the Setting of an Acute Cerebrovascular Accident

Patient not eligible for alteplase
- Systolic blood pressure (SBP) ≤220 mmHg or diastolic blood pressure (DBP) ≤120 mmHg
  ○ Observe (unless other end-organ damage present)
- SBP >220 mmHg or DBP between 121 and 140 mmHg
  ○ Aim for a 10–15% reduction in MAP
  ○ Labetolol 10–20 mg IV over 1–2 min. May repeat or double every 10 min (maximum 300 mg).
  ○ Nicardipine 5 mg/h continuous IV infusion. Titrate by 2.5 mg/h increments every 5–15 min to a maximum of 15 mg/h
- DBP >140 mmHg
  ○ Aim for a 10–15% reduction in mean arterial pressure (MAP)
  ○ Nitroprusside—0.25–0.5 mcg/kg/min continuous IV infusion; increase in increments of 0.25–0.5 mcg/kg/min until desired hemodynamic effect. Usual doses up to 2–3 mcg/kg/min. High-alert medication—read package insert before use

Patient otherwise eligible for alteplase (except for blood pressure)
- SBP >185 mmHg or DBP >110 mmHg confirmed by two consecutive measurements
  ○ Labetolol 10–20 mg IV over 1–2 min. May repeat in one dose
  ○ Nitropaste 1–2 in.
  ○ Nicardipine 5 mg/h continuous IV infusion. Titrate by 2.5 mg/h increments every 5–15 min to a maximum of 15 mg/h
  ○ If blood pressure is not *reduced* and *maintained* at target range (systolic ≤185 mmHg and diastolic ≤110 mmHg), do not administer fibrinolytic
    ▪ Aggressive treatment to reduce and maintain blood pressure excludes patients from fibrinolytic eligibility. Patients that require sodium nitroprusside to control blood pressure may not be sufficiently stable to receive fibrinolytic pharmacotherapy
  ○ Blood pressure control during and after fibrinolytic administration is SBP <180 mmHg and DBP <105 mmHg

During and after fibrinolytic therapy
- Monitor blood pressure at least every 15 min during treatment and then for another 2 h, then every 30 min for 6 h, then every hour for 16 h
- If blood pressure increases above target range
  - DBP >140 mmHg
    - Nitroprusside—0.25–0.5 mcg/kg/min continuous IV infusion; increase in increments of 0.25–0.5 mcg/kg/min until desired hemodynamic effect. Usual doses up to 2–3 mcg/kg/min. High-alert medication—read package insert before use
  - SBP >230 mmHg or DBP between 121 and 140 mmHg
    - Labetolol 10–20 mg IV over 1–2 min. May repeat or double every 10 min (maximum 300 mg). Alternatively, a continuous IV infusion (2–8 mg/min) may be initiated after the initial bolus
    - Nicardipine 5 mg/h continuous IV infusion. Titrate by 2.5 mg/h increments every 5–15 min to a maximum of 15 mg/h
    - If blood pressure not controlled, may consider nitroprusside
  - SBP between 180 and 230 mmHg or DBP between 105 and 120 mmHg
    - Labetolol 10–20 mg IV over 1–2 min. May repeat or double every 10 min (maximum 300 mg). Alternatively, a continuous IV infusion (2–8 mg/min) may be initiated after the initial bolus

Stroke 2007;38:1655–1711
Stroke 2005;36:916–921.

Table 3.3
Alteplase Inclusion and Exclusion Criteria
for Cerebrovascular Accident Indication

Inclusion criteria
- Age 18 yr or older
- Clinical diagnosis of an acute ischemic word cerebrovascular accident (CVA) causing measurable neurological deficit
- Ability to definitively establish the time of CVA onset
- Ability to begin alteplase therapy within 3 h of CVA onset
- Patient or family members understand the potential risks and benefits from treatment

Exclusion criteria

- Evidence of intracranial hemorrhage, subarachnoid hemorrhage, or a large area of cerebral edema, parenchymal hypodensities, or sulcal effacement on pretreatment CT scan
- Rapidly improving or minor symptoms
- Coma or stupor
- Active internal bleeding
- Platelet count <100,000/mm^3
- Patient is coagulopathic or has received heparin within past 48 h and has an elevated activated partial thromboplastin time (aPTT)
- Patient is coagulopathic or has recently received an oral antico-agulant (e.g., warfarin) and has an elevated international nor-malized ratio (INR) >1.4
- History of major surgery or serious trauma in the previous 14 d
- History of any intracranial or intraspinal surgery, serious head trauma, or previous CVA within previous 3 mo
- History of gastrointestinal or urinary tract hemorrhage within previous 21 d
- History of any intracranial hemorrhage
- Recent arterial puncture at a noncompressible site or biopsy within previous 7 d
- Blood pressure >185/110 mmHg on repeated measurements
- Serum glucose <50 mg/dL
- Evidence of active pericarditis, endocarditis, septic emboli, current or recent pregnancy, and lactating women
- Seizure observed at stroke onset with postictal residual neuro-logical impairments
- Acute myocardial infarction within 3 mo
- Known arteriovenous malformation, aneurysm, or intracranial neoplasm
- Head CT shows a multilobar infarction/hypodensity involving more than one-third of the cerebral hemisphere (not an absolute contraindication)
- Modified National Institute of Health Stroke Score of ≥20 (not an absolute contraindication)

Note: patients on aspirin therapy before CVA onset can still receive tPA. No recommendations are made regarding other antiplatelet agents.

Table 3.4
Modified National Institute of Health Stroke Scale

Item	Name	Response
1 A	Level of consciousness	0 = alert
		1 = drowsy
		2 = obtunded
		3 = unresponsive/coma
1 B	Orientation—2 questions (e.g., month, age)	0 = answers both correctly
		1 = answers one correctly
		2 = answers neither correctly
1 C	Commands—2 (e.g., open and close eyes)	0 = performs both tasks correctly
		1 = performs one task correctly
		2 = performs neither task
2	Gaze	0 = normal
		1 = partial gaze palsy
		2 = complete gaze palsy
3	Visual fields	0 = no visual loss
		1 = partial hemianopia
		2 = complete hemianopia
		3 = bilateral hemianopia
4	Facial palsy	0 = normal
		1 = minor
		2 = partial
		3 = compete
5	Motor function (arm)	0 = no drift
	a. Left	1 = drift before 5 s
	b. Right	2 = falls before 10 s
		3 = no effort against gravity
		4 = no movement
6	Motor function (leg)	0 = no drift
	a. Left	1 = drift before 5 s

(Continued)

Table 3.4 *(Continued)*

Item	*Name*	*Response*
	b. Right	2 = falls before 5 s
		3 = no effort against gravity
		4 = no movement
7	Limb ataxia	0 = absent
		1 = one limb
		2 = two limbs
8	Sensory	0 = normal
		1 = partial loss
		2 = severe loss
9	Language	0 = normal
		1 = mild-to-moderate aphasia
		2 = severe aphasia
		3 = mute or global aphasia
10	Dysarthria	0 = normal articulation
		1 = mild-to-moderate
		2 = severe
		9 = intubated
11	Extinction or inattention	0 = no neglect
		1 = partial neglect
		2 = complete neglect

Table 3.5
Alteplase Administration Protocol for Cerebrovascular Accident Indication

- *See* Table 3.3 for inclusion and exclusion criteria
- 0.9 mg/kg IV dose with a maximum of 90 mg
- Reconstitute with 0.9% saline
- Administer 10% of the dose intravenously over 1 min
- Administer remaining 90% of the dose intravenously over 1 h
- Admit patient to an intensive care or stroke unit for monitoring

- Monitor for changes in neurological status every 15 min during the infusion, every 30 min for the next 6 h, and then every hour until 24 h after treatment
- Monitor blood pressure every 15 min for the first 2 h, every 30 min for the next 6 h, and then every hour until 24 h after treatment. Increase frequency of monitoring if systolic blood pressure ≥180 mmHg or diastolic ≥105 mmHg
- No antiplatelet agents or anticoagulants should be administered for 24 h following the completion of alteplase (tPA) infusion
- Maintain blood pressure <180/105 mmHg for 24 h following the completion of tPA infusion
- No arterial punctures or other invasive procedures for 24 h following the completion of tPA infusion
- Discontinue infusion and obtain emergent head CT if intracranial hemorrhage is suspected (*see* Table 2.6)
- Obtain follow-up head CT at 24 h before starting antiplatelet or anticoagulant pharmacotherapy

Table 3.6
Management of an Alteplase-Induced Intracranial Hemorrhage

- Discontinue alteplase infusion immediately
- Order immediate head CT without contrast
- Check complete blood count, prothrombin time, international normalization ratio, activated partial thromboplastin time, fibrinogen levels
- If intracranial hemorrhage is confirmed, administer 5–10 units of cryoprecipitate, evaluate laboratory results, and supplement blood products and platelets as deemed necessary (e.g., 2 units fresh frozen plasma [FFP], 6–8 units platelets)
  ○ Platelet dysfunction may be seen with fibrinolytic therapy
- Evaluate patient for possible aminocaproic acid therapy
- Obtain neurosurgery consult
- Nomogram for predicting 30-d mortality[a]

[a]May be found in *Circulation* 1998;98:1376–1382.

Table 3.7
Management of Intracranial Hypertension
(Intracranial Pressure ≥20 mmHg)

General supportive measures
- Maintain cerebral perfusion pressure (CPP) between 60–80 mmHg
  - CPP = mean arterial pressure (MAP) – intracranial pressure (ICP)
  - Use fluids and/or vasopressors to elevate MAP if necessary
  - Maintain euvolemia (pulmonary capillary wedge pressure between 10 and 14 mmHg)
  - Administer pacted red blood cells (PRBCs) if HCT <30%
- Monitor for transient increases in ICP that occur with suctioning or bronchoscopy. Pretreatment with lidocaine IV may blunt this transient increase in ICP
- Seizure prophylaxis if warranted
- Adequate nutritional support
- Adequate pain control (i.e., morphine) and sedative use (i.e., propofol, benzodiazepine)
  - Effects on MAP and CPP should be monitored carefully

Interventions to decrease intracranial pressure
- Head-of-bed elevation at 30%
- Maintain patient's head in straight position
- Avoid hyperthermia
  - Use antipyretics and cooling blanket where necessary
  - Therapeutic use of hypothermia is currently not recommended
- Hyperventilate to a goal between 30 and 35 mmHg
  - Hyperventilation to 25–30 mmHg for brief periods may be considered in refractory intracranial hypertension
  - Effect limited to 24 h
  - Avoid rapid increase in CO_2 (prevent rebound)
- Mannitol (as a 15–20% solution)
  - 1 g/kg IV bolus followed by 0.25 g/kg IV q6h
  - Use in-line 5 μm filter set
  - Maintain measured serum osmolality under 310–320 mOsm/kg

- ○ Contraindicated in severe renal impairment
- ○ Effect may be limited to 24 h
- Pentobarbital coma (in refractory cases)
  - ○ Utilize a central line +/− pulmonary artery catheter
  - ○ 10 mg/kg IV over 30 min followed by 5 mg/kg/h continuous IV infusion for 3 h (total loading dose is 25 mg/kg)
  - ○ Loading dose followed by 1 mg/kg/h. Can titrate up to 3 mg/kg/h
  - ○ Slow rate if patient becomes hypotensive during the loading or maintenance infusion
  - ○ Maintain plasma levels between 30 and 40 mg/L
  - ○ Taper dose if ICP well controlled for 24–48 h
  - ○ Potent CYP 450 enzyme inducer
- Cerebrospinal fluid drain through ventriculostomy if hydrocephalus present
- Consider decompressive surgery
- No role for corticosteroids in cerebrovascular accidents or traumatic brain injury based on the available literature. May increase complication rate

Stroke 2007;38:2001–2023.
J. Neurotrauma 2000;17:449–627.

Critical Care

Table 4.1
General Drug Utilization Principles in Intensive Care

- Start with low doses and titrate carefully
- Discontinue any nonvital medication on ICU admission. Keep track of this intervention and restart medications as clinically necessary
- Review medication profile daily for drug–drug interactions
- Anticipate common drug side effects
- Avoid intramuscular route of drug administration
- Avoid the subcutaneous and intramuscular route of drug administration in patients in any form of shock
- Strict avoidance of hypoglycemia. Ensure an adequate source of dextrose in any patient receiving an insulin product
- Promote appropriate patient sleep–wake cycles
- Practice daily wake-up in patients receiving sedative medications
- Become familiar with the pharmacokinetic and pharmacodynamic principles of medications prescribed in ICU patients
- Become familiar with the principles of safe writing rules as suggested by the Institute of Safe Medication Practice
- Be aware of common sound-alike medications
- Practice good hand hygiene
- Vaccinate carefully selected patients
- Obtain and review ones institution's antibiogram

From: *Pocket Guide to Critical Care Pharmacotherapy*
By: J. Papadopoulos © Humana Press Inc., Totowa, NJ

- Always address the need for stress-ulcer prophylaxis, deep vein thrombosis (DVT) prophylaxis, anemia prophylaxis, and nutrition support

---

Table 4.2
Management of Severe Sepsis and Septic Shock[a]

Resuscitation goals during the first 6 h (early goal-directed therapy)
- Should be vigorous and titrated to clinical end points of volume repletion
- Central venous pressure between 8 and 12 mmHg
  - Use a crystalloid (normal saline or lactated Ringer's solution) or a colloid (hydroxyethyl starch or albumin 5%) intravenous boluses
    - 500–1000 mL of a crystalloid over 15–30 min and repeat as necessary
      - Up to 10 L may be required in the first 24 h
    - 300–500 mL of a colloid over 15–30 min and repeat as necessary
      - Up to 4 L may be required in the first 2 h
      - Hetastarch
        - Up to 1.5 L/d or 20 mL/kg/d
        - Contraindicated if patient has a bleeding diathesis, has hydrostatic pulmonary edema, or is anuric. Cautious use if patient is thrombocytopenic, has liver disease, or has a history of corn allergy
  - Most patients require aggressive fluid resuscitation during the first 24 h of management. Input/output ratios are not useful during this time period. Monitor for evidence of systemic or pulmonary edema
- Mean arterial pressure ≥65 mmHg
- Urine output ≥0.5 mL/kg/h
- Central venous (superior vena cava) or mixed venous oxygen saturation ≥70%
  - If goal not achieved with fluid resuscitation and the hematocrit is ≥30%, then administer dobutamine continuous IV infusion (maximum dose of 20 mcg/kg/min)

- If goal not achieved with fluid resuscitation and the hematocrit is <30%, then transfuse packed red blood cells to achieve a hematocrit ≥30%
  - Some clinicians recommend hemoglobin between 8 and 10 g/dL in patients with early septic shock (i.e., transfusion trigger of 7 g/dL). In patients with a low cardiac output, lactic acidosis, widened gastric-arterial $PaCO_2$ gradient, or significant pulmonary or cardiac disease, and a goal-directed trial to higher hemoglobin may be warranted
- A recent study would support a mixed venous oxygen saturation of 65% as similar to a central venous oxygen saturation of 70%[b]

Diagnosis
- Diagnostic studies should be performed to identify the source of infection, causative pathogen, and any complications (e.g., abscess, empyema, infected intravascular catheter, etc). A removable or drainable focus should be removed/ drained
- After appropriate cultures have been obtained, initiate appropriate spectrum empiric anti-infective therapy *within the first hour* of presentation
  - A recent trial in bacteremic septic shock showed that each hour of delay in effective antimicrobial administration over the ensuing 6 h was associated with an average decrease in survival by 7.6%[c]
- Reassess therapy after 48–72 h and continue or streamline therapy based on microbiological data, clinical response, and clinical judgment

Vasopressors
- Use when an appropriate fluid challenge fails to restore adequate hemodynamics and organ perfusion or in the face of life-threatening shock when fluid challenge is in progress. Should be utilized in patients who have been adequately fluid resuscitated
- Intravenous choices (preferably through a central venous line)
  - Norepinephrine (first-line)
    - Start with 4 mcg/min continuous IV infusion and titrate to effect. Maximum dose around 125 mcg/min or 3 mcg/kg/min

- More potent than dopamine and may be more effective in managing hypotension in septic shock
- Small studies have shown improvement in glomerular filtration rate and gastrointestinal mucosal perfusion when norepinephrine is utilized in resuscitated septic shock
○ Dopamine (first-line)
  - 2.5–20 mcg/kg/min continuous IV infusion. May require doses above 10 mcg/kg/min for an adequate response
  - Useful in patients with systolic dysfunction
  - No role for low-dose (renal) dopamine
○ Vasopressin
  - Not yet a first-line agent (the recent Vasopressin in Septic Shock Trial [VASST] showed no difference in 28-d mortality when vasopressin was compared with norepinephrine)
  - May be considered in patients with refractory septic shock
  - 0.01–0.04 units/min continuous IV infusion
    □ Doses >0.04 units/min have been associated with myocardial ischemia, decreased cardiac output, and cardiac arrest
○ Phenylephrine (second-line)
  - Start with 50 mcg/min continuous IV infusion and titrate to effect. Maximum dose around 400 mcg/min
○ Epinephrine (refractory hypotension)
  - Start with 0.05 mcg/kg/min continuous IV infusion and titrate to effect. Dose range is 2–10 mcg/min
  - Doses under 0.05 mcg/kg/min may exacerbate hypotension

Inotropes
- Potentially useful in resuscitated patients with persistent evidence of systemic or organ hypoperfusion
- Increasing cardiac index to predefined supranormal levels has not been found to improve outcome
- Dobutamine
  ○ 2.5–10 mcg/kg/min continuous IV infusion up to 20 mcg/kg/min

- ○ May cause hypotension and tachycardia
- Milrinone
  - ○ 0.2–0.75 mcg/kg/min continuous IV infusion
  - ○ Loading dose of 50 mcg/kg over 10 min may be utilized
    - ▪ Avoid or administer 50% if tenuous hemodynamics
  - ○ Use lower doses in patients with renal dysfunction (i.e., 0.2 mcg/kg/min)
  - ○ Can be used cautiously as a primary inotrope or in combination with dobutamine
  - ○ If utilized, may require starting or increased doses of a vasopressor

Corticosteroids
- The recent CORTICUS trial (hydrocortisone vs placebo) does not support the routine use of corticosteroids in the management of septic shock. No difference in 28-d mortality was observed between groups, regardless of baseline relative adrenal insufficiency. Duration of shock was shorter in the hydrocortisone group; however, an increased incidence of hyperglycemia, sepsis, and recurrent septic shock was observed. This section reflects the 2004 consensus guidelines
- Hydrocortisone 50 mg IV q6h or 100 mg IV q8h for 7 d in patients with septic shock requiring vasopressor support if relative adrenal insufficiency present
  - ○ Administer ACTH 250 mcg IV (ACTH stimulation test)
    - ▪ Check a pre-ACTH stimulation test cortisol level at 30, 60, and possibly 90 min post-ACTH administration
  - ○ If serum cortisol increase is ≤9 mcg/dL, then patient may have relative adrenal insufficiency
    - ▪ Some clinicians advocate a baseline cortisol level <15 mcg/dL[d] or <25 mcg/dL[e] in critically ill patients as the diagnostic threshold for relative (or functional) adrenal insufficiency
  - ○ Do not wait for results to initiate corticosteroid therapy if in shock
  - ○ Discontinue if patient does not have relative adrenal insufficiency
  - ○ Some clinicians advocate dose tapering after shock resolution at the end of therapy

  ○ Some clinicians would add fludrocortisone 50 mcg enterally
     daily to hydrocortisone pharmacotherapy

Drotrecogin-α (recombinant human activated protein C)
- Use based on institution-specific protocol
- Recommended in patients with a high risk of death
  ○ APACHE II score ≥25
  ○ Sepsis-induced organ dysfunction
  ○ No *absolute* contraindications present
    - Active internal bleeding
    - Recent (within 3 mo) hemorrhagic stroke
    - Recent (within 2 mo) intracranial or intraspinal surgery, or
      severe head trauma
    - Trauma with an increased risk of life-threatening bleeding
    - Presence of an epidural catheter
    - Intracranial neoplasm, mass lesion, or evidence of cerebral
      herniation
  ○ Potential benefit outweighs any relative contraindications
     present
  ○ Platelets should be maintained ≥30,000/mm^3
  ○ 24 mcg/kg/h continuous IV infusion for 96 h
    - Dose based on actual body weight (even in obese
      patients)

Glycemic control
- Recommendations in this section may change based on results
  from the recent GLUCONTROL trial and the Volume
  Substitution and Insulin Therapy in Severe Sepsis Study. Both
  trials where stopped early due to lack of efficacy and safety
  concerns.
- Maintain blood glucose between 80–110 mg/dL or
  80–150 mg/dL
  ○ Use a continuous IV infusion of insulin based on an institu-
     tion-specific protocol
  ○ Should be used with a continuous enteral or intravenous
     source of dextrose
    - Aggressively avoid and treat hypoglycemia

○ Based on the results of a recent trial, one editorialist recommends target glucose between 80–150 mg/dL for the first 3 d in the ICU. If ICU stay exceeds 3 d, a goal between 80–110 mg/dL could be considered[f]

---

[a]*NEJM* 2006;354:449–461; *Crit Care Med.* 2004;32:1928–1948; *Crit. Care Med.* 2004;32:858–873; *NEJM* 2001;345:1359–1377.
[b]*Int. Care Med.* 2004;30:1572–1578.
[c]*Crit. Care Med.* 2006;34:1589–1596.
[d]*NEJM.* 2003;348:727–734.
[e]*Crit. Care Med.* 31:141–145.
[f]*NEJM* 2006;354(5):516–517.

Table 4.3
Sedation, Analgesia, and Delirium Guidelines[a]

Sedation
- Address etiology of agitation and/or anxiety
  ○ Hypoxia, hypercarbia, pain, central nervous system infections, hypoglycemia, electrolyte imbalances, substance withdrawal, and sleep
  deprivation
    ▪ If patient is sleep deprived, consider altering the patient's environment and possibly a nighttime sedative to promote an appropriate sleep–wake cycle
- Establish predetermined end points using a sedation and agitation scale (*see* Tables 4.4 and 4.5)
  ○ The target level of sedation will be patient dependant
  ○ Bispectral index monitoring may be of some value in patients who are deeply sedated
- Optimize the environment and minimize lighting, noise, and frequent vital sign checks
- Methods of intravenous administration
  ○ Continuous IV infusion
  ○ Intermittent IV bolus
- Management of acute agitation
  ○ Midazolam 2–5 mg intravenous push (IVP) every 5–15 min

- Short-term sedative requirements (<48–72 h)
  - Midazolam 0.04–0.2 mg/kg/h continuous IV infusion
    - Active metabolite may accumulate in patients with renal impairment
  - Propofol 5–20 mcg/kg/min continuous IV infusion (preferably through a central line)
    - *Nutritional considerations:* Contains soy bean oil, egg lecithin, and glycerol. Provides 1.1 kcal/mL of emulsion; may need to adjust nutritional regimen. One formulation contains EDTA. Prolonged therapy with the EDTA-containing product may decrease serum zinc levels. May need to monitor serum zinc levels and supplement. Monitor serum triglyceride levels with prolonged infusions
    - Propofol infusion syndrome has been described and may result in severe metabolic acidosis, cardiac dysrhythmias, cardiovascular collapse, rhabdomyolysis, and death. The risk may be increased with concomitant catecholamine infusions or when the dose exceeds 80 mcg/kg/min
  - Dexmedetomidine (≤24 h) 1 mcg/kg IV for >10 min, followed by 0.2–0.7 mcg/kg/h continuous IV infusion
    - Some clinicians either omit the bolus dose or administer half the recommended amount
- Sedative requirements for >72 h
  - Convert midazolam or propofol to *lorazepam*
  - Lorazepam 0.01–0.1 mg/kg/h continuous IV infusion or 1–4 mg IV every 4–6 h
  - Propofol 5–20 mcg/kg/min continuous IV infusion (in patients who require frequent neurological assessment)
- Reassess goals daily and titrate/taper dose to desired response (as patients may accumulate the medication or become tolerant)
  - With downward titration, monitor for signs/symptoms of withdrawal
    - Anxiety, agitation, delirium, diaphoresis, myoclonus, tremors, and seizures
  - Consider daily wake-up as per hospital protocol

- The addition of a narcotic analgesic to a sedative may have additive effects. Monitor and titrate to desired level of sedation if used concomitantly
- Lorazepam may be preferred over other benzodiazepines in patients with renal and/or hepatic insufficiency

Analgesia
- Evaluate location, intensity, characteristics, and aggravating/alleviating factors
  - ○ Assess intensity by utilizing a visual analog or numeric rating scale (0–10 with 10 being the worst possible pain)
  - ○ Assess subjectively through vital signs and/or facial/body expressions if patient cannot communicate
  - ○ Establish predetermined end points
- Methods of intravenous administration
  - ○ Continuous IV infusion
  - ○ Intermittent IV bolus
  - ○ Patient-controlled analgesia in noncritically ill patients
  - ○ As needed, method (e.g., prn) should be avoided if patient has continuous analgesic requirements
- Patient hemodynamically unstable
  - ○ Fentanyl 1–3 mcg/kg/h continuous IV infusion or 25–100 mcg IVP every 5–15 min
    - ■ Less histamine release than morphine
- Patient hemodynamically stable
  - ○ Morphine 1–10 mg/h continuous IV infusion
    - ■ For acute pain administer 2–5 mg IVP every 5–15 min
    - ■ Avoid prolonged use or high doses in patients with renal failure
  - ○ Fentanyl 1–3 mcg/kg/min continuous IV infusion
    - ■ For acute pain administer 25–100 mcg IVP every 5–15 min
  - ○ Hydromorphone 7–15 mcg/kg/h or 0.5–1 mg/h continuous IV infusion
    - ■ For acute pain administer 0.25–0.75 mg IVP every 5–15 min
- Avoid meperidine, buprenorphine, butorphanol, and nalbuphine
- NSAIDs or acetaminophen may be used as adjunctive agents in the appropriate patient

- Reassess goals daily and titrate/taper dose to desired response (as patients may accumulate the medication or become tolerant)
  - With downward titration, monitor for signs/symptoms of withdrawal
    - Tachycardia, hypertension, tachypnea, mydriasis, lacrimation, diaphoresis, rhinorrhea, piloerection, vomiting, diarrhea, yawning, muscle cramps, irritability, and anxiety

Delirium
- Use the Confusion Assessment Method for the ICU (Table 4.6) to evaluate patient
- If possible, discontinue any benzodiazepines, as they may cause paradoxical agitation and delirium. Evaluate for reversible etiologies
- Drugs that may cause delirium
  - Opioids, benzodiazepines, barbiturates, corticosteroids, dopamine agonists (e.g., amantadine, bromocriptine, levodopa, pergolide, pramipexole, ropinirole), H_2-receptor antagonists, anticholinergics (e.g., diphenhydramine, trihexylphenidyl), β-adrenergic blockers, clonidine, methyldopa, carbamazepine, phenytoin, baclofen, cyclobenzaprine, lithium, antidepressants (e.g., tricyclic antidepressants, selective serotonin reuptake inhibitors), and interleukin-2
- Haloperidol 2 mg slow IVP, followed by doubling the dose every 15–20 min until desired effect. For maintenance regimen, add up total loading dose and administer 25% every 6 h for a few days. Then taper dose over several days
  - Monitor for QT-interval prolongation and extrapyramidal side effects
- Olanzapine 2.5–10 mg enterally daily may be an alternative to haloperidol. Start with 2.5 mg in elderly or debilitated patients

[a]*Crit. Care Med.* 2002;30:119–141.

Note: Critically ill patients (e.g., elderly, organic mental syndrome, pulmonary, cardiac, renal, and/or hepatic impairment) may be at increased risk for adverse drug events. Start with the lowest dose and titrate very carefully.

Table 4.4
Modified Ramsey Sedation Scale[a]

1	(awake)	Anxious and agitated or restless or both
2		Cooperative, oriented, and tranquil
3		Responds to commands only
4	(asleep)	Brisk response to a light glabellar tap or loud auditory stimulus
5		Sluggish response to a light glabellar tap or loud auditory stimulus
6		No response to a light glabellar tap or loud auditory stimulus

[a]*Br Med J.* 1974;2:656–659.

Table 4.5
Riker Sedation-Agitation Scale[a]

Score	Description	Definition
7	Dangerous agitation	Pulling at endotracheal tube (ETT), trying to remove catheters, climbing over bedrail, striking at staff, thrashing side-to-side
6	Very agitated	Does not calm despite frequent verbal reminding of limits, requires physical restraints, biting ETT
5	Agitated	Anxious or mildly agitated, attempting to sit up, calms down with verbal instructions
4	Calm and cooperative	Calm, awakens easily, follows commands
3	Sedated	Difficult to arouse, awakens with verbal stimuli or gently shaking but drifts off again, follows simple commands

(Continued)

Table 4.5 *(Continued)*

Score	Description	Definition
2	Very sedated	Arouses to physical stimuli but does not communicate or follow commands, may move spontaneously
1	Unarousable	Minimal or no response to noxious stimuli, does not communicate or follow commands

[a]*Crit. Care Med.* 1999;27:1325–1329.

Table 4.6
Confusion Assessment Method for the Diagnosis of Delirium in Intensive Care Unit Patients[a]

Features	Assessment variable
1- Acute onset of mental status changes or fluctuating course	• Is there evidence of an acute change change in mental status from baseline? • Did the abnormal behavior fluctuate during the past 24 h? • Did the sedation scale (e.g.,Riker Sedation-Agitation scale) or Glasgow coma scale fluctuate in the past 24 h?
2- Inattention	• Did the patient have difficulty focusing attention? • Is there a reduced ability to maintain and shift attention? • How does the patient score on the Attention Screening Examination (ASE)? ○ Visual component ASE tests the patient's ability to pay attention through recall of 10 pictures

(Continued)

Table 4.6 *(Continued)*

Features	Assessment variable
	○ Auditory component ASE tests attention through having patient squeeze hands or nod whenever the letter "A" is called in a random letter sequence
3- Disorganized thinking	• If the patient is already extubated from the ventilator, determine whether or not the patient's thinking is disorganized or incoherent, such as rambling or irrelevant conversation, unclear or illogical flow of ideas, or unpredictable switching from subject to subject
	• For patients still intubated, can the patient answer the following four questions correctly?
	○ Will a stone float on water?
	○ Are there fish in the sea?
	○ Does one pound weigh >2 pounds?
	○ Can you use a hammer to pound a nail?
	• Was the patient able to follow questions and commands throughout the assessment?
	○ Are you having unclear thinking?
	○ Hold up this many fingers (examiner holds up two fingers in front of the patient)
	○ Now do the same thing with the other hand (examiner not hold ing up any fingers)

(Continued)

Table 4.6 *(Continued)*

Features	Assessment variable
4- Altered level of consciousness (any level other than alert)	• Alert—normal, spontaneously fully aware of the environment, interacts appropriately • Vigilant—hyperalert • Lethargic—drowsy but easily aroused, unaware of some elements in the environment, or not spontaneously interacting appropriately with the examiner; becomes fully aware and appropriately interactive when prodded minimally • Stupor—difficult to arouse, unaware of some or all elements in the environment, or not spontaneously interactive with the examiner; becomes incompletely aware and inappropriately interactive when prodded strongly; can be aroused only by vigorous and repeat stimuli and as soon as the stimulus ceases, stuporous subjects lapse back into the unresponsive state • Coma—unarousable, unaware of all elements in the environment, with no spontaneous interaction or awareness of the examiner, so that the interview is impossible even with maximal prodding

[a]*Crit. Care Med.* 2001;29:1370–1379.

Note: Patients are diagnosed with delirium if they have both features 1 and 2 and either 3 or 4.

Table 4.7
Neuromuscular Blocker Use in the Intensive Care Unit

Indications
- Facilitate endotracheal intubation
  - Succinylcholine 1–1.5 mg/kg IV up to 150 mg total dose
  - Contraindications may include use in patients with a personal or family history of malignant hyperthermia, extensive/severe burns, myopathies with elevated creatine phosphokinase, penetrating eye injuries, pre-existing hyperkalemia, narrow-angle glaucoma, and disorders of plasma pseudocholinesterase
- Facilitate mechanical ventilation
  - Decrease oxygen consumption
- Control increased intracranial pressures
- Control muscle spasm associated with tetanus

Sedation and analgesic pharmacotherapy must be optimized before the use of neuromuscular blockade (NMB)
- NMBs *does not* possess sedative, amnestic, or analgesic properties

If the patient is adequately sedated and there is still a need for NMB then:
- Pancuronium
  - 0.05–0.1 mg/kg IV bolus followed by 1 mcg/kg/min continuous IV infusion once recovery from bolus is observed
  - Adjust dose for renal dysfunction
  - Use another NMB if contraindications exist to vagolytic activity (i.e., cardiovascular disease)
- Cisatracurium or atracurium in the presence of renal and/or hepatic dysfunction
  - Cisatracurium
    - 0.15–0.2 mg/kg IV bolus followed by 3 mcg/kg/min continuous IV infusion once recovery from bolus dose is observed. Usual dose range between 0.5 and 5 mcg/kg/min.
  - Atracurium

- ▪ 0.4–0.5 mg/kg IV bolus followed by 9–13 mcg/kg/min continuous IV infusion once recovery from bolus dose is observed
- Consider daily discontinuation of NMB and patient assessment if prolonged infusions are required
- Try a different NMB if tachyphylaxis develops to one NMB

Monitor
- Train-of-four
  - ○ Superficial nerves
    - ▪ Ulnar nerve—monitor response of the adductor pollicis (thumb)
    - ▪ Posterior tibial nerve—monitor flexion of the big toe and foot
    - ▪ Facial nerve—monitor contraction of the orbicularis oculi muscle
  - ○ Target number of twitches depends on patient's condition and depth of sedation
    - ▪ Usually goal is 1/4 or 2/4 twitches
  - ○ Percent receptor occupation and resultant NMB:
    - ▪ 3/4 twitches—80% receptor occupation
    - ▪ 2/4 twitches—85% receptor occupation
    - ▪ 1/4 twitches—85–90% receptor occupation
    - ▪ 0/4 twitches—90–95% receptor occupation
- Clinical status and respiratory effort
- Visual and tactile assessment of muscle tone
- Clinical evidence of undersedation
  - ○ Tachycardia, hypertension, piloerection, and diaphoresis
- Bispectral index (BIS) monitor
- Muscle weakness and damage
  - ○ Check periodic creatine phosphokinase levels with prolonged infusions (especially if patient is receiving concomitant corticosteroid pharmacotherapy)
    - ▪ Try to avoid this drug combination

Preventative strategies
- Appropriate deep vein thrombosis (DVT) prophylaxis
- Reposition patient as appropriate to prevent decubitus ulcer formation

- Ophthalmic ointment, drops, or taping the eyelids shut to prevent keratitis and corneal abrasion

---

aCrit Care Med. 2002;30:142–156.

Table 4.8
Reversal of Nondepolarizing Neuromuscular Blockers

Combination IV agents	Dose when 3/4 TOF	Dose when 2/4 TOF	Dose when 1/4 TOF
Edrophonium + Atropine	10 mg **(0.5–1 mg/kg)** + 7–14 mcg/kg	10 mg **(0.5–1 mg/kg)** + 7–14 mcg/kg	Do not use
Neostigmine + Glycopyrrolate	0.5–1 mg **(0.04 mg/kg [5 mg maximum])** + 5 mcg/kg	1–1.5 mg **(0.07 mg/kg [5 mg maximum])** + 10 mcg/kg	2–2.5 mg **(0.08 mg/kg [5 mg maximum])** + 15 mcg/kg
Pyridostigmine + Glycopyrrolate	0.1 mg/kg + 5 mcg/kg	0.2 mg/kg + 10 mcg/kg	0.3 mg/kg + 15 mcg/kg

Notes:

1. TOF—train-of-four
2. Postpone reversal until a twitch is observed
3. Administer anticholinergic agent 1–2 min before acetylcholinesterase inhibitor
4. Doses are estimated based on recommended dosing ranges and TOF
   a. There is considerable difference of opinion regarding optimum dosage. In general, anesthesiology literature/references recommend higher doses *(the bold text reflects anesthesia literature recommendations)*. Consult a clinician with expertise in this field in a situation of uncertainty.
5. Up to 60-min time to recovery with a long-acting neuromuscular blocker (i.e., pancuronium, doxacurium)
6. Up to 30-min time to recovery with an intermediate-acting neuromuscular blocker (i.e., atracurium, cisatracurium, rocuronium, and vecuronium)

Table 4.9
Factors that Alter the Effects of Neuromuscular Blockers

Increase effect	*Decrease effect*
Clinical	*Clinical*
• Hypokalemia, hypocalcemia, hyponatremia, hypermagnesemia	• Alkalosis
• Acidosis, hypothermia	• Hypercalcemia
• Renal failure	• Demyelinating lesions
• Hepatic failure	
• Neuromuscular diseases	
Medications	*Medications*
• Anesthetics	• Anticholinesterases
○ Desflurane, enflurane, isoflurane, halothane	• Calcium
• Antimicrobials	• Carbamazepine, phenytoin
○ Aminoglycosides, clindamycin, polymyxins, vancomycin	• Theophylline, caffeine
• Class I Antiarrhythmics	
• β-adrenergic blockers	
• Calcium channel blockers	
• Dantrolene	
• Lithium	

Table 4.10
Management of Malignant Hyperthermia[a]

Triggers
- Volatile inhalational anesthetics
  - ○ Desflurane, enflurane, halothane, isoflurane, and sevoflurane
- Succinylcholine

Management
- Discontinue offending agent
- Stabilize airway, breathing, and circulation
- Hyperventilate with 100% oxygen
- Dantrolene IV

- ○ 2.5 mg/kg IV every 5–10 min as necessary up to a maximum of 10 mg/kg
- ○ Followed by 1–2 mg/kg enterally every 6 h for 72 h
- Cool patient
  - ○ Evaporative cooling
    - Patient is repeatedly wetted down by sponging or spraying the skin with tepid water while a fan is blowing air across the body service
  - ○ The effectiveness and safety of strategic ice packing (groin, axillae), whole body ice packing, and gastric or peritoneal lavage is controversial
  - ○ Cooling efforts should continue until the core body temperature reaches 38°C or 100.4°F
  - ○ Shivering (a common complication of cooling, which can add to heat generation) can be managed with:
    - Meperidine 25–50 mg IV in one dose. Cautious use in patients with hepatic or renal disease or seizure predisposition
    - Lorazepam 1–2 mg IV q 4–6 h prn
  - ○ There is no role for acetaminophen or aspirin antipyretic pharmacotherapy
- Maintain intravascular volume status and urine output with normal saline
  - ○ Add furosemide as needed
- Manage complications:
  - ○ Rhabdomyolysis, arrhythmias, seizures, and disseminated intravascular coagulation (DIC)

*[a]*www.mhaus.org.

Table 4.11
Use of Packed Red Blood Cell Transfusions and Erythropoietin in Critically Ill Patients[a]

Potential adverse effects of packed red blood cell (PRBCs) transfusions
- Immediate immunological complications

- ○ Anaphylactic/anaphylactoid reactions, transfusion-related acute lung injury (TRALI), hemolysis, platelet destruction, and fever
- Delayed immunological complications
  - ○ Alloimmunization to red cells, white cells, and platelets
    - ■ Delayed hemolytic reactions
  - ○ Graft vs host disease
- Transfusion-related immunomodulation (TRIM)
- Hypothermia
- Infectious
  - ○ Viral
    - ■ Hepatitis B and C, HIV 1 and HIV 2, cytomegalovirus, HTLV I and HTLV II, and West Nile virus
  - ○ Bacterial
    - ■ *Yersinia enterocolitica*, *Babesia* spp., *Bartonella* spp., *Borrelia* spp., and *Brucella* spp.
  - ○ Others
    - ■ *Leishmania* spp., *Rickettsia*, *Parvovirus* spp., plasmodia and *Toxoplasma* spp., and prions
- Iron overload
- Metabolic complications
  - ○ Hypocalcemia (owing to citrate binding)
  - ○ Hyperkalemia
  - ○ Metabolic alkalosis (citrate hepatically metabolized to bicarbonate)
- Volume overload (TACO—transfusion-associated cardiac overload)

Establish institution-specific erythropoietin guidelines with transfusion thresholds. Transfusion guidelines and triggers should account for an individual patient's ability to tolerate and compensate for an acute decrease in hemoglobin, based on signs and symptoms of impaired global and regional tissue oxygenation

Suggestions for the appropriately identified patient:
- Pacted red blood cells (PRBCs)
  - ○ Controversy exists regarding the appropriate transfusion trigger

- ○ Hemoglobin trigger <7 g/dL in most intensive care unit patients
  - ■ Goal between 7 and 9 g/dL
- ○ Hemoglobin trigger <10 g/dL in patients with:
  - ■ A significant cardiac history *and* evidence of current ischemia
  - ■ Acute hemorrhage
  - ■ Goal above 10 g/dL
  - ■ Further studies needed in this group
- Expected duration of ICU stay of >3–7 d
  - ○ Erythropoietin (epoetin-alpha)
  - ○ Recommendations in this section may change based on the results from the recent EPO-3 trial (epoetin alfa versus placebo). A difference in red blood cell transfusion rates was not observed between groups. Epoetin alpha therapy improved survival in trauma patients. Epoetin alfa did not have a measurable clinical benefit in medical/surgical non-trauma patients. Epoetin alpha therapy was associated with an increased thrombotic event rate, particularly in patients not receiving pharmacological deep vein thrombosis prophylaxis.
    - ■ 40,000 units SQ once weekly for 3–4 doses
    - ■ Potential alternative may be darbepoetin 100 mcg SQ once weekly
    - ■ Initiate on ICU day three
    - ■ Consider intravenous administration in patients in distributive shock
      - ▫ The optimal intravenous dosing regimen is not known
      - ▫ Intravenous administration displays a different pharmacokinetic profile than subcutaneous administration
    - ■ May take several weeks to observe a pharmacological response
  - ○ Iron therapy
    - ■ Require between 150 and 200 mg elemental iron per day for adequate erythropoiesis (e.g., ferrous sulfate 325 mg enterally TID provides 195 mg of elemental iron)

---

[a]*JAMA* 2002;288:2827–2835; *NEJM* 1999;340:409–417.

Table 4.12
Propylene Glycol Content of Commonly Utilized
Intravenous Medications[a]

Chordiazepoxide	207 mg/mL
Conivaptan	300 mg/mL
Diazepam	414.4 mg/mL
Digoxin	414.4 mg/mL
Esmolol (2.5 g/10 mL ampule)	250 mg/mL
Etomidate	350 mg/mL
Hydralazine	103.6 mg/mL
Lorazepam (2 mg/mL)	830 mg/mL
MVI-12 (adult)	310.8 mg/mL
Nitroglycerin	310–518 mg/mL
Pentobarbital	414.4 mg/mL
Phenobarbital	702.4 mg/mL
Phenytoin	414.4 mg/mL
Trimethoprim/sulfamethoxazole	414.4 mg/mL

[a]*Int. Care Med.* 2002;28:81–84.

Note:

1. Chronic or large ingestions of propylene glycol have been associated with the development of hyperosmolar anion-gap metabolic acidosis, renal dysfunction, hemolysis, cardiac arrhythmias, and seizures.
2. Monitor osmolar gap in patients receiving prolonged or high doses of above intravenous medications (e.g., lorazepam ≥10 mg/h infusion for >48 h).
3. A toxic propylene glycol plasma level breakpoint remains to be determined.
4. Propylene glycol is partially excreted by the kidney unchanged and partially metabolized by hepatic alcohol dehydrogenase to lactic acid and pyruvate.
5. Must evaluate volume of medication administered to determine total propylene glycol exposure. High-dose lorazepam (i.e., >8–10 mg/h), phenytoin loading doses, and phenobarbital are the most likely offenders.

Table 4.13
Drug-Induced Fever

- Etiology probably multifactorial (i.e., hypersensitivity reactions, pharmacological action of the drug and/or metabolites, infusion-related, altered thermoregulation, idiosyncratic)
- Rash, urticaria, visceral organ abnormalities, and peripheral eosinophilia may be seen
- Fever pattern may range in severity and perserverance; may cause a pulse-temperature deficit.
- Resolution of fever may occur 72 h after the discontinuation of the offending agent

Medications
- Abacavir
- Allopurinol
- Anticholinergic agents (e.g., antihistamines, atropine, tricyclic antidepressants)
- Aspirin (severe overdose)
- Barbiturates, carbamazepine, and phenytoin (antiepileptic hypersensitivity syndrome)
- Bleomycin
- Amphotericin B, cephalosporins, penicillins, minocycline, nitrofurantoin, sulfonamide antimicrobials, and vancomycin
- Heparin
- Hydralazine, methyldopa, procainamide, and quinidine
- L-asparaginase, immunoglobulins, and interferons
- Jarisch-Herxheimer reaction following treatment of syphilis, brucellosis, schistosomiasis, or trypanosomiasis
- Malignant hyperthermia (*see* Table 4.10)
- Neuroleptic malignant syndrome (*see* Table 12.2)
- Serotonin syndrome (*see* Table 12.3)
- Vaccines
- Zonisamide

- Altered thermoregulation
  - Atropine, antihistamines, phenothiazines, and haloperidol
  - Amphetamines, cocaine, and ecstasy (methylene dioxymethamphetamine)
- Intravenous infusion-associated
  - Amphotericin B, bleomycin, and pentazocine

Table 4.14
Pharmaceutical Dosage Forms That Should not be Crushed

- Any extended release preparation
  - CR—controlled-release
  - EC—enteric coated
  - LA—long-acting
  - SR—sustained release
  - TR—time release
  - SA—sustained action
  - SL—sublingual
  - XL—extended length
  - XR—extended release

Table 4.15
Stress-Related Mucosal Damage Prophylaxis Protocol

Assess patient for the presence of risk factors
- Mechanical ventilation for >48 h
- Coagulopathy (i.e., thrombocytopenia or disseminated intravascular coagulation)
- Septic shock
  - Systolic blood pressure (SBP) <90 mmHg or a mean arterial pressure (MAP) <60 mmHg for >1 h or hypotension requiring vasopressor pharmacotherapy
- Head or spinal cord injury

- Major trauma
- Major surgery
- Burns (thermal injury) in >30% of body surface area
- Renal failure
- Liver failure
- High-dose corticosteroid therapy (e.g., hydrocortisone 200 mg/d or greater or its equivalent)

Suggested utilization guidelines
- Lack of enteral access
  - Intravenous H_2-receptor antagonist (preferred) or intravenous proton pump inhibitor (PPI)
- Presence of an NGT or PEG or patient can take PO
  - Enterally administered H_2-receptor antagonist, sucralfate, or PPI
- Presence of a transpyloric feeding tube
  - H_2-receptor antagonist or PPI
- Convincing evidence on the efficacy of enteral nutrition in the prevention of stress-related mucosal damage not available

Dosing and administration guidelines
- H_2-receptor antagonists (adjust all doses for renal impairment)
  - Famotidine: 20 mg IV or enterally q12h
  - Ranitidine: 150 mg enterally q12h or 50 mg IV q6h
  - Nizatidine: 150 mg enterally q12h
  - Cimetidine: 300 mg IV or enterally q6h
- Proton pump inhibitors (consider q12h dosing for better pH control)
  - Omeprazole: 20–40 mg enterally daily
  - Esomeprazole: 20–40 mg enterally daily or q12h
  - Lansoprazole: 30 mg enterally or IV daily
  - Pantoprazole: 40 mg enterally or IV daily or 12h
  - Rabeprazole: 20 mg enterally daily
- Sucralfate 1 g enterally q6h

- ○ May be preferred in patients whose risk of hospital-acquired pneumonia (HAP) is greater than upper gastrointestinal bleed. Data suggests a lower incidence of HAP when compared with H_2-receptor antagonist
- ○ May be less effective than H_2-receptor antagonist pharmacotherapy
- ○ Contains 207 mg aluminum/1 g. Avoid chronic use in patients with renal failure
- ○ Does not alter gastric pH

End points of prophylaxis
- Gastric pH between 3.5 and 5
  - ○ Monitor gastric pH in high-risk patients whereby possible
    - ■ Does not apply to sucralfate pharmacotherapy
  - ○ Adjust dose accordingly if gastric pH is above or below the therapeutic range
  - ○ If patient is receiving continuous enteral nutrition:
    - ■ Hold enteral nutrition for 2 h
    - ■ Flush feeding tube with 30 mL water or saline
    - ■ Obtain gastric pH after 1 h

Duration of prophylaxis
- Reassess patient daily for the presence or absence of risk factors
- Consider discontinuing prophylaxis when the patient is discharged from the intensive care unit or if risk factors abate

Table 4.16
Therapeutic Drug Monitoring

Medication	Goal steady-state levels

Amikacin	• High concentration (once-daily)
	  ○ Peak—50–60 mcg/mL
	  ○ Trough—undetectable
	• Pneumonia (standard dosing)
	  ○ Peak—25–30 mcg/mL
	  ○ Trough—4–5 mcg/mL
	• Bacteremia (standard dosing)
	  ○ Peak—20–25 mcg/mL
	  ○ Trough—4–5 mcg/mL

(Continued)

Table 4.16 *(Continued)*

Medication	Goal steady-state levels

	• Urinary tract infection (standard dosing)
	  ○ Peak—15–16 mcg/mL
	  ○ Trough—3–4 mcg/mL
	• Goal peak = 8–12 × MIC pathogen
	• Obtain peak 30–60 min after a dose
	• Obtain trough 30 min before a dose

Carbamazepine	• 4–12 mcg/mL • Obtain trough concentrations for routine monitoring
Digoxin	• Chronic heart failure—0.8–1 ng/mL • Atrial fibrillation—1.5–2 ng/mL • May check a level 4 h after an IV dose or 6 h after an enteral dose • Obtain trough concentrations for routine monitoring

Gentamicin	• High concentration (once daily)
	  ○ Peak—18–20 mcg/mL
	  ○ Trough—undetectable
	• Pneumonia (standard dosing)
	  ○ Peak—8–10 mcg/mL
	  ○ Trough—1 mcg/mL
	• Bacteremia (standard dosing)
	
	  ○ Peak—5–8 mcg/mL
	  ○ Trough—1 mcg/mL
	• Urinary tract infection (standard dosing)
	  ○ Peak—5 mcg/mL
	  ○ Trough—1 mcg/mL
	• Endocarditis (standard dosing)
	  ○ Peak—3–5 mcg/mL
	  ○ Trough—1 mcg/mL

(Continued)

Table 4.16 *(Continued)*

Medication	Goal steady-state levels
	• Goal peak = 8–12 × MIC pathogen
	• Obtain peak 30–60 min after a dose
	• Obtain trough 30 min before a dose
Lidocaine	• 1–5 mcg/mL
	• Check a level if therapy is continued beyond 24 h or if a patient has LV dysfunction or hepatic impairment
	• Has two active metabolites that are renally cleared
Phenobarbital	• 15–40 mcg/mL
	• Levels obtained within 1–2 wk after the initiation of therapy do not reflect steady-state concentrations
	• Once steady-state is achieved, levels can be obtained irrespective of when the dose is administered
Phenytoin/ Fosphenytoin	• 10–20 mcg/mL
	○ 1–2 mcg/mL for free drug
	• Some patients may need levels up to 25 mcg/mL
	• Time to achieve steady-state may be prolonged
	• May obtain a level 2 h after an IV load to assess the adequacy of the dose, then again within 2–3 d
	• May obtain a level 4 h after an IM load with fosphenytoin
	• Obtain trough concentrations for routine monitoring
	• Equation to adjusted measured phenytoin levels in the setting of hypoalbuminemia

(Continued)

Table 4.16 *(Continued)*

Medication	Goal steady-state levels
	○ Adjusted phenytoin level = measured phenytoin level/ $(0.2 \times$ serum albumin) + 0.1
	• Equation to adjust measured phenytoin levels in the setting of CrCl ≤10 mL/min (+/− hypoalbuminemia)
	○ Adjusted phenytoin level = measured phenytoin level/ $(0.1 \times$ serum albumin) + 0.1
	○ May need to monitor free phenytoin levels
Theophylline	• 5–15 mcg/mL
	• Levels above 15 mcg/mL can predispose a patient to toxicity
	• Obtain a level 24 h after the initiation of a continuous IV infusion, then daily until stable
	• Obtain trough concentrations for routine monitoring of enteral products
	• Has active metabolites that are renally cleared
Tobramycin	• High concentration (once daily)
	○ Peak—18–20 mcg/mL
	○ Trough—undetectable
	• Pneumonia (standard dosing)
	○ Peak—8–10 mcg/mL
	○ Trough—1 mcg/mL
	• Bacteremia (standard dosing)
	○ Peak—5–8 mcg/mL
	○ Trough—1 mcg/mL
	• Urinary tract infection (standard dosing)

(Continued)

Table 4.16 *(Continued)*

Medication	Goal steady-state levels
	○ Peak—5 mcg/mL
	○ Trough—1 mcg/mL
	• Goal peak = 8–12 × MIC pathogen
	• Obtain peak 30–60 min after a dose
	• Obtain trough 30 min before a dose
Valproic acid	• 50–100 mcg/mL
	• Obtain trough concentrations for routine monitoring
Vancomycin	• Pneumonia and meningitis
	○ Trough—15–20 mcg/mL
	• Other indications
	○ Trough—10–15 mcg/mL
	• Obtain trough 30 min before a dose

LV, left ventricular; MIC, mean inhibitory concentration; IV, intravenous; IM, intramuscular.

Table 4.17
Select Antidotes for Toxicological Emergencies

Acetylcysteine (NAC)
- Used in acetaminophen intoxication
- IV dose
  - 150 mg/kg over 60 min, followed by 50 mg/kg over 4 h, followed by 6.25 mg/kg/h for 16 h. Total dose is 300 mg/kg over 21 h
  - Alternative IV regimen: 140 mg/kg followed in 4 h by 70 mg/kg q4h × 17 additional doses
- Enteral dose
  - 140 mg/kg followed in 4 h by 70 mg/kg q4 h × 17 additional doses. Repeat any enteral dose if patient vomits within 1 h of administration
- Treatment duration may vary based on clinical presentation
  - Consider a longer course if treatment is delayed beyond 8 h of ingestion
- Use IV product with caution in patients with a history of asthma

Digibind

- Used in cardiac glycoside intoxication. The information below pertains to digoxin intoxication
- Indications:
  - Life-threatening dysrhythmia
  - Digoxin level ≥10 ng/mL
  - Ingestion of ≥10 mg
  - Potassium level >5 mEq/L (secondary to digoxin toxicity)
  - Lower thresholds in elderly patients
- IV dose (3 different methods to determine the number of vials in the setting of digoxin intoxication)
  - (serum concentration in ng/mL × body weight in kg)/100
- Based on steady-state levels
  - (Milligrams ingested × 0.8)/0.5
  - Acute ingestion—10–20 vials or chronic ingestion—3–6 vials
  - If 20 vials is chosen as the dose for acute ingestion, may administer in two divided doses
  - Round vial number up to the nearest vial
- Use 0.22 μm inline filter
- Administer over 30 min
  - May bolus if critically ill
- Plasma levels not useful after administration. Monitor the patient clinically
- Monitor for rebound toxicity in patients with renal impairment
- Monitor for CHF exacerbation and hypokalemia
- Contraindicated if known hypersensitivity to sheep products

Flumazenil

- Used in benzodiazepine, zaleplon, and zolpidem intoxications
- Indications:
  - Central nervous system depression with normal vital signs and normal electrocardiogram
- Avoid use if:
  - Seizure history
  - Chronic benzodiazepine use
  - Concomitant TCA intoxication
  - Concomitant arrhythmogenic or epileptogenic ingestant

- ○ Use carefully in patients with known alcohol dependence or panic attacks
- Dose (for suspected overdose)
  - ○ 0.2 mg over 30 s. If still lethargic, give 0.3 mg over 30 s. May administer 0.5 mg every 60 s to a maximum cumulative dose of 3 mg. Patients with a partial response to 3 mg may need additional titrated doses up to 5 mg. Consider an alternative diagnosis if the patient does not respond to 5 mg. May initiate a continuous IV infusion of 0.1–1 mg/h in the event of resedation (benzodiazepine half-life longer than flumazenil's half-life)
- Does not reliably reverse respiratory or cardiac depression
- Monitor for rebound benzodiazepine intoxication

Glucagon
- Used in β-adrenergic blocker and calcium channel blocker intoxication
- Dose
  - ○ 2–10 mg IV bolus followed by 3–10 mg continuous IV infusion
- Monitor for tachyphylaxis
- Methylene blue (*see* Table 8.3)

Naloxone
- Used in narcotic intoxication. Limited efficacy in clonidine intoxication
- Dose
  - ○ 0.4–2 mg IV over 30 s every 2–3 min as needed to a maximum dose of 10 mg. Use 0.1–0.2 mg increments or lower doses in opioid-dependant patients, patients with cardiovascular disease, or if the clinical situation is not life threatening. Consider an alternative diagnosis if the patient does not respond to a 10 mg dose. May initiate a continuous IV infusion at 2/3 the reversal dose in patients who experience rebound toxicity (narcotic half-life longer than naloxone's half-life)
- Use with caution in patients with cardiovascular disease or acute pulmonary edema

- Monitor for signs of opioid withdrawal in opioid-dependant patients

Octreotide
- Used in sulfonylurea and quinine intoxication (secondary after glucose administration)
- Dose
  - 50 mcg IV q4h or 50 mcg SQ q6h
  - Role for continuous IV infusion?
- Monitor for hypoglycemia and hyperglycemia

Protamine sulfate
- Used in unfractionated heparin (UFH) and low molecular weight heparin (LMWH) intoxication
  - Fully reverses UFH
  - Reverses approx 60% LMWH
- Dose
  - UFH—1 mg protamine/100 units UFH
    - Must estimate amount of UFH in circulation (use a 60 min half-life)
    - Example
      - Patient on UFH 1000 units/h continuous IV infusion has major bleeding. Method to estimate UFH burden:
        - From the previous hour—1000 units remaining
        - From 2 h ago—500 units remaining
        - From 3 h ago—250 units remaining
        - Total estimated circulating UFH that needs to be reversed = 1750 units
        - Dose of protamine = 17.5 mg
  - Enoxaparin—1 mg of protamine/1 mg enoxaparin to a maximum of 50 mg
    - If aPTT prolonged 2–4 h after the first dose, may administer an additional 0.5 mg/1 mg if required
    - Dose may depend on the lapsed time after LMWH administration (e.g., 0.5 mg protamine per 1 mg enoxaparin to a maximum of 50 mg if greater than 8 h has passed since the last administered dose)

- ○ Dalteparin or tinzaparin—1 mg protamine/100 units dalteparin or tinzaparin to a maximum of 50 mg
  - ■ If aPTT prolonged 2–4 h after the first dose, may administer an additional 0.5 mg/100 units if required
  - ■ Dose may depend on the lapsed time after LMWH administration (e.g., 0.5 mg protamine per 100 units dalteparin or tinzaparin to a maximum of 50 mg if >8 h has passed since the last administered dose)
- ○ Maximum single dose is 50 mg in any 10-min period
  - ■ Weak anticoagulant when excessively dosed (decreases factor VII levels). May have an antiplatelet effect
- ○ Administer dose slowly over 10 min
- • Risk factors for an adverse event
  - ○ Previous protamine exposure (e.g., during coronary artery bypass graft, or NPH insulin products containing protamine zinc)
  - ○ Fish allergy (salmon)
- • Monitor for heparin rebound (may occur within 8–18 h)

Pyridoxine (see *Table 10.1*)
Sodium nitrite followed by sodium thiosulfate
- • Used in cyanide (including from sodium nitroprusside) intoxication
  - ○ Dose of sodium nitrite is 300 mg or 4–6 mg/kg IV over 2 min. 150 mg or 50% of the previous dose may be given if signs of cyanide toxicity reappear
  - ○ Dose of sodium thiosulfate is 12.5 g or 150–200 mg/kg IV over 2 min. 6.25 g or 50% of the previous dose may be given if signs of cyanide toxicity reappear
- • The purpose of sodium nitrite (or amyl nitrite in the absence of IV access) is to produce methemoglobin, which binds cyanide with greater affinity than mitochondrial cytochromes. In the presence of decreased oxygen carrying capacity, as in combined exposures to cyanide and carbon monoxide (e.g., some fires), sodium nitrite can be detrimental and should be avoided.

Hydroxocobalamine (Cyanokit®)
- Used in cyanide poisonings
  - 5 g IV over 15 min. In severe poisonings and based on clinical response, a second dose of 5 g may be administered over 15 min to 2 h.

Vitamin K_1 (*see* Table 2.16)

---

aPTT, activated partial thrombin time; CHF, congestive heart failure; IV, intravenous; SQ, subcutaneous; NPH, TCA.

5

Dermatology

Table 5.1
Drug-Induced Dermatological Reactions

Angioedema
- Angiotensin converting enzyme inhibitors, atracurium, β-lactams, heparin, iron (parenteral), losartan, and streptokinase

Erythema multiforme/Stevens–Johnson syndrome/toxic epidermal necrolysis
- Allopurinol, barbiturates, carbamazepine, cephalosporins, cyclophosphamide, ethambutol, fluconazole, ibuprofen, lamotrigine, macrolides, nitrofurantoin, penicillins, phenytoin, propranolol, quinolones, sulfonamide antimicrobials, sulindac, tetracyclines, thiazides, valproic acid, and vancomycin

Maculopapular eruptions
- Allopurinol, barbiturates, benzodiazepines, captopril, carbamazepine, erythromycin, fluoroquinolones, isoniazid, NSAIDs, penicillins, phenothiazines, phenytoin, rifampin, sulfonamides antimicrobials, and tetracyclines

Photosensitivity reactions
- Amantadine, amiodarone, barbiturates, benzodiazepines, carbamazepine, chlorpromazine, fluoroquinolones, furosemide, NSAIDs, promethazine, psoralens, quinidine, simvastatin, sulfonamide antimicrobials, sulfonylureas, tetracyclines, and thiazides

From: *Pocket Guide to Critical Care Pharmacotherapy*
By: J. Papadopoulos © Humana Press Inc., Totowa, NJ

Skin discoloration
- Blue—amiodarone (blue-gray), FD&C dye no. 1, and methylene blue
- Red—anticholinergic agents (e.g., antihistamines, atropine, tricyclic antidepressants, scopalamine), disulfiram, hydroxocobalamin, and vancomycin
- Yellow—β-carotene

Systemic lupus erythematosis
- Atenolol, hydralazine, procainamide, quinidine, carbamazepine, chlorpromazine, ethosuximide, isoniazid, methyldopa, minocycline, penicillamine, phenylbutazone, phenytoin, thiazides, and valproic acid

Urticaria
- Albumin, aminophylline, aspirin, heparin, insulin, metoclopramide, NSAIDs, muromonab-CD3 (OKT3), opiates, penicillins, propafenone, quinidine, senna, sulfonamide antimicrobials, and vancomycin

6

Endocrinology

Table 6.1
Management of Diabetic Ketoacidosis

- Identify precipitating factors
  - Infection, acute coronary syndrome, cerebrovascular accidents, trauma, noncompliance with insulin pharmacotherapy, new onset diabetes mellitus, and medications (e.g., corticosteroids and sympathomimetics)
- Prepare a comprehensive flow sheet with vitals, laboratory data, fluid type and rates, insulin rates, and other treatment
- Correct fluid abnormality
  - One liter normal saline rapidly, then 1 L/h × 2 h, then 150–300 mL/h
    - The optimal infusion rate is dependent on the volemic and hemodynamic status of the patient
    - Monitor for hyperchloremic metabolic acidosis
  - If serum sodium rises more than 150 mEq/L or when euvolemic, switch to hypotonic fluid replacement. Lactated Ringer's solution may prolong ketoacid production by promoting alkalinization
    - Serum sodium may rise with insulin and isotonic saline fluid administration. Estimate the corrected serum sodium concentration at presentation
      - Add 1.6 mEq/L to the measured serum sodium for every 100 mg/dL rise in serum glucose >200 mg/dL

From: *Pocket Guide to Critical Care Pharmacotherapy*
By: J. Papadopoulos © Humana Press Inc., Totowa, NJ

- ○ When plasma glucose falls to <250 mg/dL, switch to D5W, D5W/half NS, or D5W/NS depending on plasma sodium concentration
- Regular insulin
  - ○ Correct hypokalemia (withhold insulin bolus until repletion is underway)
  - ○ Prepare 100 units of insulin in 100 mL normal saline
  - ○ 10 units or 0.1 units/kg IV bolus, then 0.05–0.1 units/kg/h continuous IV infusion
    - Consider withholding insulin bolus in the setting of shock until resuscitation is underway. Rapid lowering of serum glucose can precipitate worsening hypovolemia
  - ○ Increase to 0.1–0.2 units/kg/h if no improvement in hyperglycemia within 2–4 h
  - ○ When plasma glucose drops to 250 mg/dL, decrease insulin infusion rate and continue until acidosis is corrected (i.e., anion gap closes)
    - Maintain plasma glucose between 200 and 250 mg/dL during the first 6–10 h, then between 150 and 200 mg/dL
  - ○ Monitor plasma glucose every 1–2 h
    - The combined effect of fluids and insulin should decrease plasma glucose by approx 100–200 mg/dL per hour
    - If hypoglycemia develops in the setting of continued ketoacidosis, lower the insulin infusion and administer glucose infusions to maintain euglycemia. Do not stop the insulin infusion
  - ○ Monitor anion gap as often as necessary
- Convert to insulin glargine (Lantus®) or NPH SQ insulin (several methods depending on style) once ketoacidosis has resolved and the patient is eating
- Monitor and correct potassium, phosphorus, and magnesium
  - ○ Potassium levels may decrease with therapy
- Bicarbonate therapy (if desired)
  - ○ No proven benefit except for concomitant symptomatic hyperkalemia
  - ○ Goal is to increase the pH >7.2
  - ○ Administer half ampule (22 mEq) if arterial pH is <7.1

- ○ Administer one ampule (44 mEq) if arterial pH is <7.0
- ○ Monitor arterial or venous pH hourly
- ○ Do not overcorrect pH as acetoacetate and β-hydroxybutyrate are metabolized to bicarbonate
- Administer all intravenous medications in saline where possible
- Monitor for evidence of cerebral edema, noncardiogenic (permeability) pulmonary edema, acute respiratory distress syndrome, hyperchloremic metabolic acidosis, and vascular thrombosis

---

Table 6.2
Management of Hyperglycemic Hyperosmolar Nonketotic Syndrome

- Identify precipitating factors
    - ○ Infection, acute coronary syndrome, cerebrovascular accidents, and trauma
- Prepare a comprehensive flow sheet with vitals, laboratory data, fluid type and rates, insulin rates, and other treatment
- Correct fluid abnormality
    - ○ Restore intravascular volume with normal saline if in hypovolemic shock
    - ○ Then/or 2–3 L of half NS over first 2 h
        - ■ The optimal infusion rate is dependent on the clinical status of the patient and choice of crystalloid
        - ■ Monitor for hyperchloremic metabolic acidosis
        - ■ Estimate the corrected serum sodium concentration at presentation
            - □ Add 1.6 mEq/L to the measured serum sodium for every 100 mg/dL rise in serum glucose >200 mg/dL
    - ○ Calculate free water deficit
        - ■ Administer half of this volume as half NS over the next 12 h
        - ■ Administer the remaining volume as half NS over the next 24 h

- ○ When plasma glucose falls to <250 mg/dL, switch to D5W or D5/half NS depending on plasma sodium concentration
- Regular insulin
  - ○ Correct hypokalemia
  - ○ Prepare 100 units of insulin in 100 mL half NS
  - ○ 10 units or 0.1 units/kg IV bolus, then 0.05 units/kg/h continuous IV infusion
    - Patients with hyperglycemic hyperosmolar nonketotic syndrome may require less insulin than DKA for acute glycemic control
  - ○ Increase to 0.1 units/kg/h if no improvement in hyperglycemia within 2–4 h
  - ○ When plasma glucose drops to 250 mg/dL, decrease insulin infusion rate and continue
    - Maintain plasma glucose between 200 and 250 mg/dL during the first 6–10 h, then between 150 and 200 mg/dL
    - Maintain infusion for 24–36 h
  - ○ Monitor plasma glucose every 1–2 h
- Convert to insulin glargine (Lantus®) or NPH SQ insulin (several methods depending on style) once glycemic control is achieved and the patient is eating
- Monitor and correct potassium, phosphorus, and magnesium
- Administer all intravenous medications in half NS as appropriate
- Monitor for evidence of cerebral edema, noncardiogenic (permeability) pulmonary edema, acute respiratory distress syndrome, hyperchloremic metabolic acidosis, and vascular thrombosis

---

Table 6.3
Management of Thyrotoxic Crisis and Myxedema Coma

Thyrotoxic crisis
- Supportive care
  - ○ Control hyperthermia with acetaminophen and cooling blanket

- Avoid aspirin, as it may increase free T_4 and T_3 levels by interfering with plasma–protein binding
  ○ Fluid resuscitation
- Propylthiouracil (preferred thionamide, as it blocks peripheral conversion of $T_4 \rightarrow T_3$)
  ○ 200 mg enterally every 4–6 h. Reduce dose once signs/symptoms are controlled. Usual maintenance dose is 100–150 mg q8h
  ○ Alternative—methimazole 30 mg enterally every 6–8 h. Reduce dose once signs/symptoms are controlled. Usual maintenance dose is 15–60 mg daily in three equally divided doses
- Lugol's solution 10 drops or 1 mL in water q8h
  ○ Alternative—saturated solution of potassium iodide (SSKI) 5–10 drops in water q8h
  ○ Use iodine solutions at least 1–2 h after a thionamide
  ○ If the patient is iodine allergic, can administer lithium carbonate 300 mg enterally q6h to achieve a plasma level around 1/L
- β adrenergic blockers
  ○ Adjust dose to achieve heart rate ≤100 beats/min
  ○ Cautious use in setting of heart failure related to systolic dysfunction
  ○ Propranolol 0.5–1 mg slow intravenous push (IVP) up to a total of 5 mg, then 20–80 mg enterally q6h
  ○ Esmolol may be utilized if a rapid short-acting agent is needed
- Hydrocortisone 100 mg IV q8h or 50 mg IV q6h until adrenal suppression is excluded. Also blocks peripheral conversion of $T_4 \rightarrow T_3$
- Consider plasmapheresis if intractable symptoms

Myxedema coma
- Supportive care
  ○ Rewarm passively with a blanket. Active rewarming may cause distributive shock

- ○ Treat hypotension with fluids and vasopressor support. Consider adrenal insufficiency
- ○ Manage hyponatremia if present
- Levothyroxine (T_4) 200–500 mcg IV bolus followed by 75–100 mcg/d
  - ○ Reduce dose in patients with coronary artery disease
- Liothyronine (T_3) 25–50 mcg IV bolus. Use 10–20 mcg IV bolus in patients with CAD. Subsequent doses (e.g., 2.5–10 mcg IV q6-8h) should be administered between 4–12 h after the initial bolus dose and continued until signs and symptoms resolve
- Role for dual T_3 and T_4 therapy is uncertain
- Hydrocortisone 100 mg IV q8h or 50 mg IV q6h until adrenal insufficiency is excluded
- Low threshold for empiric antimicrobial therapy

7

Gastrointestinal

Table 7.1
Management of Acute Nonvariceal Upper Gastrointestinal Bleeding[a]

Address etiology

Risk factors for rebleeding

- Clinical
  - Prolonged hypotension
  - Age >65 yr
  - Fresh blood in emesis, in nasogastric aspirate, or on rectal examination
  - Evidence of active bleeding
  - Large transfusion requirements
  - Low initial hemoglobin
  - Coagulopathic
  - Concomitant diseases (e.g., hepatic, renal, and neoplasm)
- Endoscopic
  - Ulcers >1–2 cm in size
  - Site of bleeding
    - Posterior lesser gastric curvature or posterior duodenal wall
  - Evidence of stigmata of recent hemorrhage
    - Spurting vessel
    - Oozing vessel
    - Nonbleeding visible vessel (NBVV)
    - Ulcer with an adherent clot

From: *Pocket Guide to Critical Care Pharmacotherapy*
By: J. Papadopoulos © Humana Press Inc., Totowa, NJ

Management
- Appropriate fluid resuscitation
- Placement of a nasogastric tube in the appropriate patient
  - Benefits may include
    - Potential reduction in risk of massive aspiration if placed initially in an awake patient
    - Facilitates endoscopic view
    - May help gauge activity and severity of bleeding
- Urgent endoscopy (within 24 h of presentation)
- Histamine$_2$-receptor antagonists are *not* recommended
- Pantoprazole IV
  - In patients with evidence of stigmata of recent hemorrhage
  - May be initiated prior to endoscopy
  - 80 mg IV over 2 min followed by 8 mg/h continuous IV infusion for up to 72 h
  - Step down to oral/enteral proton pump inhibitor (high dose) once stable (e.g., esomeprazole 40 mg bid or pantoprazole 40 mg bid)
  - Esomeprazole or lansoprazole may be utilized as alternative intravenous agents
- Oral/enteral proton pump inhibitor
  - In patients with a flat spot or clean ulcer base
- Octreotide 50 mcg IV bolus followed by 50 mcg/h continuous IV infusion for 3–5 d
  - In patients with evidence of a spurting or oozing vessel who are at the highest risk of rebleeding (personal opinion)[b]
- *Helicobacter pylori* testing and treatment when appropriate

[a]*Ann. Intern. Med.* 2003;139:843–857.
[b]*Ann. Intern. Med.* 1997;127:1062–1071.

Table 7.2
Causes of Diarrhea in the Intensive Care Unit Patient[a]

Medications
- Antimicrobials (noninfectious)
- Sorbitol-containing solutions
  - Guaifenesin, theophylline, and valproic acid

- Prokinetic agents
  - Metoclopramide and erythromycin
- Histamine$_2$-receptor antagonists, proton pump inhibitors, magnesium-containing enteral products, and misoprostol
- Digoxin, procainamide, and quinidine

Enteral nutrition formulas (especially hyperosmotic formulas)

Infectious
- *Clostridium difficile, Staphylococcus aureus,* and *Candida* spp.
- Uncommon—*Salmonella* spp., *Shigella* spp., *Campylobacter* spp., *Yersinia* spp., and enteropathogenic *Escherchia coli*

Others
- Fecal impaction, ischemic bowel, pancreatic insufficiency, and intestinal fistulae
- Gastrointestinal neoplasm
  - Vasoactive intestinal polypeptide secreting tumors

[a]*Am. J. Gastroenterol.* 1997;92:1082–1091; *Hepatology* 1998;27:264–272.

Table 7.3
Managing the Complications of Cirrhosis

Supportive measures
- Abstinence from alcohol
  - Alcohol withdrawal prophylaxis or treatment
- Nutrition support
  - Protein restriction should not be routinely utilized
- Corticosteroid therapy for patients with alcoholic hepatitis (steatonecrosis) with or without hepatic encephalopathy
  - Maddrey score or discriminant function = 4.6 (patient's prothrombin time – prothrombin time control) + total bilirubin
    - If the score is ≥32 and/or patient is encephalopathic, consider administering prednisone or prednisolone (the active form of prednisone) if there is no evidence of an upper gastrointestinal tract hemorrhage or an active infection
  - 6 wk of prednisone or prednisolone taper

- Example, 40 mg enterally bid × 1 wk, 40 mg enterally daily × 1 wk, 20 mg enterally daily × 2 wk, and 10 mg enterally daily × 2 wk. Alternative regimen is 40 mg enterally daily for 4 wk followed by a taper
- More data on etanercept, infliximab, and pentoxifylline are needed before any recommendations can be made

Ascites (serum ascites albumin gradient > 1.1 g/dL)
- Reduced sodium intake (≤2 g/d)
- Fluid restriction not necessary unless serum sodium <120–125 mEq/L
- Diuretics
  - Spironolactone 50–200 mg enterally daily
  - Furosemide 20–80 mg enterally daily
    - Monitor for excessive diuresis
  - 100 mg spironolactone/40 mg furosemide ratio to maintain normokalemia. Doses may be adjusted every 3–5 d up to a maximum of spironolactone 400 mg per day and furosemide 160 mg per day. Single morning doses increase patient compliance
  - Amiloride may be a less effective alternative to spironolactone
    - 5–20 mg/d
  - Once edema has resolved, maintenance weight loss should not exceed 0.5 kg per day
  - Stop diuretic pharmacotherapy if serum creatinine acutely rises >2 mg/dL, patient becomes encephalopathic, or serum sodium of <120 mEq/L despite fluid restriction

Tense ascites
- Large-volume paracentesis
  - If removing >5 L of fluid, consider albumin volume expansion to prevent hemodynamic compromise, rapid reaccumulation of ascites, dilutional hyponatremia, or hepatorenal syndrome (controversial)
    - Replace with 8–10 g albumin/L of ascitic fluid removed
  - Avoid large-volume paracentesis in patients with pre-existing hemodynamic compromise, acute renal insufficiency, active infection, or active upper gastrointestinal bleed. Cautious large-volume paracentesis in patients with tense

ascites *and* respiratory compromise or evidence of abdominal compartment syndrome
- High-dose diuretics until loss of ascitic fluid
  - Spironolactone up to 400 enterally daily
  - Furosemide up to 160 enterally daily

Refractory ascites
- Serial therapeutic paracentesis (as above under tense ascites)
- Transjugular intrahepatic porto-systemic shunt (TIPS)
- Peritoneovenous shunt
- Liver transplantation

Hepatic encephalopathy (acute)
- Precipitating factors
  - Infection, constipation, metabolic alkalosis, hypokalemia, excessive dietary protein intake, gastrointestinal hemorrhage, hypoxia, and hypovolemia
  - Drugs with sedative properties (e.g., benzodiazepines)
    - Management
  - Address precipitating factors
  - Protein restriction in patients with grade III or IV hepatic encephalopathy
    - Limit to 40 g/d or 0.5 g/kg/d whereas providing appropriate nonprotein calories
      - Add protein back in 20 g increments every 3–5 d once acute hepatic encephalopathy improves and until protein caloric goal is achieved (usually 0.8–1 g/kg/d)
    - Specialized enteral formulas may have a role in carefully selected patients
      - Nutrihep, hepatic-aid, and hepatamine (IV)
    - Vegetable protein better tolerated than animal protein
      - Contains less aromatic amino acids
  - Lactulose
    - 30–60 mL enterally every 1–2 h until defecation, then 15–30 mL q6h titrated to achieve 2–3 soft stools per day
    - In NPO patients, a retention enema can be utilized
      - 300 mL lactulose syrup in 700 mL water held for 30–60 min q6-8h

- ○ Neomycin 0.5–1 g enterally q6h
  - Duration should be ≤2 wk to avoid systemic accumulation and renal toxicity
- ○ Lactulose + neomycin combination therapy if inadequate response to lactulose monotherapy
- ○ Metronidazole 500 mg enterally q8h can be a substitute for neomycin
- ○ Limited experience with rifaximin 400 mg enterally q8h
- ○ Zinc sulfate 220 mg enterally q8-12h (efficacy questionable)
  - Zinc is a cofactor for ammonia metabolism
  - Presence of malnutrition and diarrhea can lead to zinc deficiency

Hepatorenal syndrome—type 1 (rapid, progressive decline in renal function)

- Avoid NSAIDs and nephrotoxins
- Assess patient for prerenal azotemia and hold diuretic therapy
  - ○ Fluid resuscitate if evidence of volume depletion
- In patients with spontaneous bacterial peritonitis
  - ○ Albumin IV 1.5 g/kg on day 1, then 1g/kg on day 3
- Consider midodrine 7.5 mg enterally q8h + octreotide 100 mcg SQ q8h
  - ○ Administer with concomitant albumin volume expansion
    - 1 g/kg IV on day 1, followed by 20–40 per day
    - Titrate to appropriate volume status and central venous pressure
  - ○ Goal is to increase mean arterial pressure (MAP) by 15 mmHg
    - Can increase midodrine to a maximum of 12.5 mg enterally q8h
    - Can increase octreotide to a maximum of 200 mcg SQ q8h
    - Can use octreotide in combination with phenylephrine in patients without enteral access
  - ○ Duration of therapy is 5–20 d
  - ○ End point of therapy
    - Decrease serum creatinine to <1.5 mg/dL
- Consider large-volume paracentesis if evidence of abdominal compartment syndrome is secondary to tense ascites
- Liver transplantation

Spontaneous bacterial peritonitis (SBP)

Treatment
- Albumin IV 1.5 g/kg on day 1, then 1 g/kg on day 3 to decrease renal failure and mortality
- Antimicrobial pharmacotherapy usually for 7–10 d
  - ○ Should target *Enterobacteriaceae* and *streptococci*
  - ○ β-lactam/β-lactamase inhibitor combinations, third or fourth-generation cephalosporins, or a fluoroquinolone
  - ○ Must inquire about previous antimicrobial use and evaluate for bacterial resistance

Secondary pophylaxis
- Long-term daily fluoroquinolone or trimethoprim/sulfamethoxazole

Primary prophylaxis
- Risk factors
  - ○ Low ascitic fluid protein level (≤1 g/dL) or serum total bilirubin >2.5 mg/dL
  - ○ Either short-term inpatient therapy or long-term daily therapy with either a fluoroquinolone or trimethoprim/sulfamethoxazole

Variceal hemorrhage
- Secure airway
- Fluid resuscitation (avoid hypervolemia)
- Low threshold for invasive monitoring
- Emergent endoscopy
  - ○ Band ligation
  - ○ Sclerotherapy
    - ▪ Ethanolamine, sodium tetradecyl sulfate, sodium morrhuate, and polidocanol
- Antimicrobial prophylaxis if ascites/cirrhosis present preferably before endoscopy
  - ○ β-lactam/β-lactamase inhibitor combinations, third or fourth-generation cephalosporin, trimethoprim/sulfamethoxazole, or a fluoroquinolone for 7 d

- Octreotide 50 mcg IV, followed by 50 mcg/h continuous IV infusion for 5 d
  - Consider tapering infusion on day 5 to prevent rebound increase in splanchnic pressures
- Vasopressin + nitroglycerin IV *(octreotide preferred pharmacotherapy)*
  - Vasopressin 0.2–0.8 units/min
  - Nitroglycerin counteracts systemic vasoconstrictive effects of vasopressin
- Pantoprazole IV *(questionable benefit)*
  - 80 mg IV over 2 min followed by 8 mg/h continuous IV infusion for up to 72 h
  - Step down to oral/enteral proton pump inhibitor once stable
  - Esomeprazole or lansoprazole may be alternative intravenous agents
- Endoscopic refractory cases
  - Balloon tamponade followed by TIPS or surgical portosystemic shunt may be indicated
- Secondary prophylaxis[a]
  - Propranolol or nadolol
    - Increase dose until the heart rate decreases by 25% or to 55–60 bpm
    - Dose propranolol carefully in patients with a TIPS procedure because of increased enteral bioavailability
  - Endoscopic monitoring with intervention every 1–2 wk until varix/varices has/have healed, then every 3–6 mo
  - Evaluate for liver transplantation
- Balloon tamponade
- TIPS

---

[a]Detailed recommendations in *NEJM* 2001;345(9):669–681.

Table 7.4
Drug-Induced Hepatotoxicity[a]

Autoimmune
- Diclofenac, fenofibrate, lovastatin, methyldopa, minocycline, nitrofurantoin, phenytoin, and propylthiouracil

Cholestasis
- Amiodarone, ampicillin, amoxicillin, captopril, chlorpromazine, ceftriaxone, erythromycin estolate, estrogen products, methimazole, nafcillin, rifampin, sulfonamide antimicrobials, and sulfonylureas

Fibrosis
- Amiodarone, methotrexate, methyldopa, and hypervitaminosis A

Hepatocellular damage
- Acetaminophen, bosentan, diclofenac, isoniazid, lovastatin, methyldopa, niacin, nefazodone, phenytoin, propylthiouracil, rifampin, trazodone, valproic acid, and venlafaxine

Immunoallergic reactions
- Allopurinol, amoxicillin/clavulanic acid, dicloxacillin, erythromycin derivatives, halothane, phenytoin, and trimethoprim/sulfamethoxazole

Steatonecrosis
- Alcohol, amiodarone, didanosine, l-asparaginase, piroxicam, stavudine, tamoxifen, tetracycline derivatives, valproic acid, and zidovudine

Veno-occlusive disease
- Azathioprine, cyclophosphamide, nicotinic acid, tetracycline, and vitamin A

[a]*NEJM* 203;349:474–485.

Table 7.5
Drug-Induced Pancreatitis

Allergic
- Angiotensin converting enzyme inhibitors, azathioprine, mercaptopurine, mesalamine, sulfasalazine, sulfonamide antimicrobials, and tetracyclines

Direct toxic effect
- Didanosine, l-asparaginase, lamivudine, metformin, pentamidine, statins, stavudine, sulindac, valproic acid, and zalcitabine

Hypertriglyceridemia mediated
- Estrogens, furosemide, hydrochlorothiazide, interferon alfa-2b, isotretinoin, propofol, and protease inhibitors (e.g., indinavir, nelfinavir, ritonavir, and saquinavir)

Spasm of the sphincter of Oddi
- Octreotide, and opiates

8

Hematology

Table 8.1
Drug-Induced Hematological Disorders

Agranulocytosis
- β-lactam antimicrobials, chloramphenicol, chloroquine, clindamycin, dapsone, doxycycline, flucytosine, ganciclovir, isoniazid, metronidazole, nitrofurantoin, pyramethamine, rifampin, streptomycin, sulfonamide antimicrobials, vancomycin, and zidovudine
- Acetazolamide, captopril, ethacrynic acid, furosemide, hydralazine, methazolamide, methyldopa, procainamide, thiazide diuretics, and ticlopidine
- Allopurinol, aspirin, carbamazepine, chlorpropamide, clomipramine, clozapine, colchicine, desipramine, gold salts, imipramine, levodopa, penicillamine, phenothiazines, phenytoin, propylthiouracil, and sulfonylureas

Aplastic anemia
- Acetazolamide, allopurinol, aspirin, captopril, carbamazepine, chloramphenicol, chlorpromazine, dapsone, felbamate, gold salts, metronidazole, methimazole, penicillamine, pentoxifylline, phenothiazines, phenytoin, propylthiouracil, quinidine, sulfonamide antimicrobials, sulfonylureas, and ticlopidine

Hemolysis (oxidative)
- Benzocaine, β-lactams, chloramphenicol, chloroquine, dapsone, hydroxychloroquine, methylene blue, nitrofurantoin, phenazopyridine, rasburicase, and sulfonamide antimicrobials

From: *Pocket Guide to Critical Care Pharmacotherapy*
By: J. Papadopoulos © Humana Press Inc., Totowa, NJ

Hemolytic anemia
- β-lactam antimicrobials, gatifloxacin, indinavir, isoniazid, levofloxacin, nitrofurantoin, ribavirin, rifabutin, rifampin, silver sulfadiazine, streptomycin, sulfonamide antimicrobials, and tetracyclines
- Acetazolamide, amprenavir, captopril, hydralazine, hydrochlorothiazide, methyldopa, procainamide, quinidine, ticlopidine, and triamterene
- Levodopa, methylene blue, phenazopyridine, quinine, and tacrolimus

Megaloblastic anemia
- Azathioprine, chloramphenicol, colchicine, cyclophosphamide, cytarabine, 5-fluorodeoxyuridine, 5-fluorouracil, hydroxyurea, mercaptopurine, metformin, methotrexate, phenobarbital, phenytoin, primidone, proton pump inhibitors, pyrimethamine, sulfasalazine, and vinblastine

Methemoglobinemia
- Benzocaine, cetacaine, EMLA cream, lidocaine, prilocaine, and procaine
- Chloroquine, dapsone, methylene blue (doses ≥4 mg/kg), nitrofurantoin, phenazopyridine, primaquine, rasburicase, and sulfonamide antimicrobials
- Nitrates (e.g., amyl nitrate and nitroglycerin) and nitroprusside

Thrombocytopenia
- Amphotericin B products, β-lactam antimicrobials, isoniazid, linezolid, rifampin, sulfonamide antimicrobials, and vancomycin
- Abciximab, aminophylline, amiodarone, amrinone, aspirin, carbamazepine, chlorpromazine, danazol, diltiazem, eptifibatide, heparin, histamine$_2$-receptor antagonists, low molecular weight heparins, methyldopa, milrinone, procainamide, quinidine, quinine, NSAIDs, thiazide diuretics, ticlopidine, tirofiban, and valproic acid

---

NSAID, nonsteroidal anti-inflammatory drugs.

Table 8.2
Management of Heparin-Induced Thrombocytopenia[a]

- Discontinue all heparin and low molecular weight heparin sources
  - Intravenous, subcutaneous, flushes, and heparin-coated catheters
- Monitor for evidence of thrombosis
- Avoid low molecular weight heparins (high cross-reactivity)
- Avoid warfarin monotherapy during the acute phase of heparin-induced thrombocytopenia (HIT)
  - Has been associated with paradoxical venous limb gangrene and skin necrosis. If warfarin has been initiated at the time HIT is recognized, reverse with vitamin K_1 (5–10 mg enterally or IV)
- Avoid platelet transfusions
- Aspirin and inferior venacaval filters are not considered adequate therapies
- Pharmacotherapy
  - Direct thrombin inhibitors (DTIs) for a minimum of 7 d or until the platelet count has risen to normal values
    - Argatroban 2 mcg/kg/min continuous IV infusion
      - Monitor activated partial thromboplastin time (aPTT) 2 h after the start of the continuous infusion
      - Decrease dose in patients with hepatic impairment. Read package insert before use
    - Lepirudin 0.4 mg/kg IV bolus, followed by 0.15 mg/kg continuous IV infusion
      - Monitor aPTT 4 h after the start of the continuous infusion
      - Decrease dose in patients with renal impairment. Read package insert before use
      - Antibodies develop in 30% after initial and 70% after repeat exposure. Fatal anaphylaxis has been reported after sensitization
    - Alternative agents
      - Bivalirudin: Used as an alternative to heparin during cardiopulmonary bypass in patients with a history if HIT
      - Fondaparinux
      - Danaparoid (10% cross-reactivity)
        - Not available in the United States
  - Avoid interruptions of pharmacotherapy

- Ultrasonography of the lower limbs
- Conversion to warfarn and duration of therapy
  - HIT with or without evidence of thrombosis
    - Convert to oral warfarin pharmacotherapy once the platelet count has returned to baseline values (preferably >100–150 × 10^9/L). Continue for at least 30 d in patients without evidence of thrombosis (optimal duration is not known but one author recommends at least 2–3 mo of warfarin (*Blood*, 2003). Continue for at least 6 mo in patients with evidence of thrombosis
      - Determine baseline international normalized ratio (INR) and aPTT on DTI monotherapy
      - Start with warfarin ≤5 mg dose
      - Identify the desired INR target (e.g., 1.5–2 point increase)
      - Avoid overshooting target INR. Small doses of vitamin K may be administered if a patient develops a supratherapeutic INR[c]
    - Overlap with parenteral therapy for a minimum of 4–5 d or until the INR has been in the therapeutic range for *two* consecutive days
    - After the desired overlap and target INR has been reached, withhold the DTI and recheck the INR and aPTT in 4–6 h. Prolonged cessation may be required if the patient initially required a low-dose DTI infusion. If the INR is between 2 and 3 and the aPTT is at/near baseline, the DTI can be discontinued.
      - The argatroban package insert advises overlapping with warfarin aiming for an INR ≥4. Once achieved, check package insert for direction
  - Further anticoagulation may be required based on original indication for heparin
    - Duration as per indication

[a]*Chest* 2004;126:311S–337S.

[b]*Blood* 2003;101(1):31–37.

[c]*Chest* 2005;127:27S–34S; *Ann. Int. Med.* 1997;127:804–812.

Table 8.3
Management of Methemoglobinemia

Determine etiology
- Medications
  - Benzocaine, cetacaine, EMLA cream, lidocaine, prilocaine, and procaine
  - Chloroquine, dapsone, methylene blue (doses ≥4 mg/kg), nitrofurantoin, phenazopyridine, primaquine, rasburicase, and sulfonamide antimicrobials
  - Nitrates (e.g., amyl nitrate and nitroglycerin) and nitroprusside
- Chemical agents
  - Aniline dyes, antipyrine, benzene derivatives, chlorates, and chlorobenzene
  - Dinitrophenol, dinitrotoluene, trinitrotoluene, naphthalene, and nitric oxide
  - Paraquat, phenol, and silver nitrate
  - Smoke inhalation
- Foods high in nitrates or nitrites
- Well water contaminated with fertilizer (nitrates)
- Hereditary
  - NADH methemoglobin reductase deficiency
  - Hemoglobin M (histidine replaced with tyrosine in heme)

Management of acquired methemoglobinemia
- Supportive care
  - Oxygen, intubation if necessary
  - Decontamination if indicated
- Action level is patient-specific
  - ≥20% methemoglobin level in symptomatic patients
  - ≥30% methemoglobin level in asymptomatic patients
  - Patients with heart disease, pulmonary disease, central nervous system disease, or anemia should be treated at lower methemoglobin thresholds
  - Conversion rate (with removal of offending agent) of methemoglobin back to hemoglobin is about 15%/h
- Withdrawal of offending agent

- Dextrose infusion
  - Needed for NADH and NADPH synthesis (Emden-Meyerhof and hexose monophosphate shunt pathway, respectively)
- Methylene blue
  - 1–2 mg/kg IV over 5 min
    - Flush with 15–30 mL of normal saline
    - Repeat dose of 1 mg/kg IV for over 5 min in 30–60 min if needed
    - Cooximetry cannot be used to follow initial response, because methylene blue is detected as methemoglobin
  - Use cautiously in patients with known G6PD deficiency
    - May precipitate a Heinz body hemolytic anemia or methemoglobinemia
    - May be ineffective, as NAPDH is required to convert methylene blue to leukomethylene blue (reducing agent)
    - Lower doses (i.e., 0.3–0.5 mg/kg increments) may be utilized with careful monitoring in life-threatening situations
- Adjunctive pharmacotherapy in dapsone-induced methemoglobinemia
  - Cimetidine 300 mg IV or enterally q6h
    - Duration depends on dapsone half-life (~20–30 h but prolonged with cimetidine use) and methemoglobin levels
    - Prevents formation of hydroxylamine (oxidizing) metabolite of dapsone
  - Ascorbic acid has a questionable role
- Blood transfusions may be indicated with methemoglobin levels ≥50% and evidence of tissue hypoxia

Causes of an inadequate response to methylene blue
- Persistent effects of oxidizing agent
- G6PD deficiency
- Presence of sulfhemoglobinemia
- NADH methemoglobin reductase deficiency
- Presence of hemoglobin M

Management
- Exchange transfusions?
- Hyperbaric oxygen therapy?

Ann. Emerg. Med. 1999;34:646–656.

9

Infectious Disease

Table 9.1
Common Causes of Fever in Intensive Care Unit Patients

- Pneumonia
- In-dwelling catheters
- Pressure sores
- *Clostridium difficile* colitis
- Sinusitis (in patients with a nasogastric tube)
- Acalculous cholecystitis
- Pancreatitis
- Venous thromboembolism
- Drug fever (refer to Table 4.12)

Table 9.2
Prevention of Hospital-Acquired and Ventilator-Associated Pneumonia

Nonpharmacological
- Avoid tracheal intubation if possible
- Avoid nasal intubation
- Removal of nasogastric and endotracheal tubes when appropriate
- Shorten duration of mechanical ventilation
- Avoid gastric overdistention (<150 mL)
- Subglottic suctioning (questionable efficacy)
- Drain ventilator circuit condensate

From: *Pocket Guide to Critical Care Pharmacotherapy*
By: J. Papadopoulos © Humana Press Inc., Totowa, NJ

- Use of heat and moisture exchangers
- Avoid unnecessary ventilator circuit changes/manipulation
  ○ Unless visually contaminated with blood, emesis, or purulent secretions
- Semirecumbent positioning (between 30 and 45°, even during patient transport)
- Maintain appropriate endotracheal cuff pressure
- Formal infection control program
- Appropriate hand washing and/or use of ethanol-based hand sanitizers
  ○ Note that the ethanol-based hand sanitizers are not sporicidal

Pharmacological
- Avoid unnecessary antimicrobials
- Short-course antimicrobials
- Avoid unnecessary stress to ulcer prophylaxis that alters gastric pH
  ○ Sucralfate does not alter gastric pH
- Vaccinations in the appropriate patients
  ○ *Streptococcus pneumonia*, *Haemophilus influenzae*, and influenza virus
- Avoid unnecessary red blood cell transfusions

Crit. Care Med. 2004;32:1396–1405.

Table 9.3
Management of Hospital-Acquired and Ventilator-Associated Pneumonia

- Obtain appropriate cultures and sensitivities
- Calculate clinical pulmonary infection score (refer to Table 9.4)
- Early invasive diagnosis of ventilator-associated pneumonia (VAP) utilizing either broncho-alveolar lavage or protected specimen brush techniques may improve outcome by facilitating identification of a causative pathogen or facilitating diagnosis of extrapulmonary infections
- Initiate early, aggressive, and empiric intravenous therapy

- ○ Target all likely organisms
  - Must know common prevalent organisms and resistance patterns in your institution and intensive care unit
- ○ Early-onset hospital-acquired pneumonia
  - Occurring 2–4 d after acute care hospital admission
  - Commonly associated with antibiotic-sensitive bacteria
  - *Streptococcus pneumoniae, Haemophilus influenzae,* and *oxacillin-sensitive Staphylococcus aureus*
    - □ Unless risk factors for infection owing to potentially antibiotic-resistant bacteria
- ○ Late-onset hospital-acquired pneumonia
  - Occurring ≥5 d after acute care hospital admission
  - Usually antibiotic-resistant bacteria
  - Oxacillin-resistant *S. aureus, Pseudomonas aeruginosa, Acinetobacter* spp., *Enterobacter* spp., and *Klebsiella pneumoniae*
- ○ Ventilator-associated pneumonia
  - Nosocomial bacterial pneumonia developing in patients on mechanical ventilation
  - *Early-onset* (within 48–72 h after mechanical intubation)
    - □ Antibiotic-sensitive bacteria
    - □ Unless risk factors for infection owing to potentially antibiotic-resistant bacteria
  - *Late-onset* (>72 h after mechanical intubation)
    - □ Antibiotic-resistant bacteria
    - □ Oxacillin-resistant *S. aureus, P. aeruginosa, Acinetobacter* sp., *Enterobacter* sp., and *K. pneumoniae*
- • Antimicrobial pharmacotherapy (combination therapy)
  - ○ Oxacillin-resistant *S. aureus* coverage
    - Vancomycin
      - □ Target trough levels between 15 and 20 mcg/mL (to increase pulmonary penetration)
    - Linezolid
      - □ In patients who have received a recent course of vancomycin and/or are critically ill (based on a high APACHE II score)
  - ○ Broad Gram-negative coverage including *P. aeruginosa*

- ▪ Recommend initial combination therapy to increase probability of having at least one drug that covers the likely pathogen (personal opinion)
- ▪ Piperacillin-tazobactam, cefepime, imipenem, or meropenem *plus either*:
  - ▫ An aminoglycoside (consider high-concentration [once-a-day] dosing in patients with a creatinine clearance above 30 mL/min) *or*
  - ▫ Ciprofloxacin (400 mg IV q8h and adjust for creatinine clearance) or levofloxacin (750 mg IV qd and adjust for creatinine clearance)
- Stream-line antimicrobial therapy based on clinical judgment, patient response, and microbiological data
- Consider short-course therapy (8 d) based on clinical judgment and patient response
  - ○ May not apply to pneumonias caused by *P. aeruginosa* or *Acinetobacter* spp.

Am. J. Resp. Crit. Care Med. 2005;171:388–416.
Drugs 2003;63(20):2157–2168.
Chest 2002;122:2183–2196.
JAMA 2003;290:2588–2598.

Table 9.4
Clinical Pulmonary Infection Score (CPIS) Calculation

Temperature (°C)
- 36.5 – 38.4 = 0 points
- 38.5 – 38.9 = 1 point
- >39 or <36 = 2 points

Blood leukocyte count (mm³)
- 4000 – 11,000 = 0 points
- <4000 or >11,000 = 1 point
- Bands >50%, add 1 additional point

Tracheal secretions
- Absent = 0 points
- Nonpurulent = 1 point
- Purulent = 2 points

Oxygenation (PaO_2/FIO_2 in mmHg)
- >240 = 0 points
- Presence of ARDS = 0 points
- ≤240 = 2 points

Pulmonary radiography
- No infiltrate = 0 points
- Diffuse or patchy infiltrate = 1 point
- Localized infiltrate = 2 points

Progression of pulmonary infiltrate
- No progression = 0 points
- Radiographic progression = 2 points
  - Exclude ARDS and pulmonary edema

Tracheal aspirate cultures (semiquantitative analysis of pathogenic bacteria)
- No growth, rare or light quantity = 0 points
- Moderate or heavy quantity = 1 point
- Same pathogenic bacteria seen on Gram-stain, add 1 additional point

Am. J. Resp. Crit. Care Med. 2000;162:505–511.
Am. Rev. Resp. Dis. 1991;143:1121–1129.

Note:
(a) CPIS score >6 is the threshold for suspected pneumonia.
(b) At baseline, assess the first five variable, and
(c) At 72 h, assess all seven variables.

10

Neurology

Table 10.1
Management of Convulsive Status Epilepticus

Identify etiology
- Cerebrovascular accident (CVA), subarachnoid hemorrhage (SAH), intracerebral hemorrhage (ICH), central nervous system (CNS) tumor, head trauma, CNS infection, and pre-eclampsia/eclampsia
- Low antiepileptic drug levels, drug overdose (e.g., cocaine, isoniazid, theophylline, phenothiazine), ethanol-related, and drug withdrawal
- Cerebral hypoxia/anoxia, hypoglycemia, hyponatremia, hypernatremia, hypomagnesemia, hypocalcemia, and hypercalcemia (rare)

Management
- Airway/breathing/circulation (ABCs)
- Oxygen by nasal cannula or mask
  - Consider endotracheal intubation if respiratory assistance is needed
- Obtain appropriate laboratory tests
  - Complete blood count, serum chemistries, arterial blood gases, and antiepileptic blood levels
  - Urine and blood toxicological panel
- Manage complications
  - Hyperthermia, metabolic acidosis, arrhythmias, cerebral edema, and rhabdomyolysis

From: *Pocket Guide to Critical Care Pharmacotherapy*
By: J. Papadopoulos © Humana Press Inc., Totowa, NJ

- Thiamine (unless patient is known to be euglycemic)
  - 100 mg IV in one dose administered *before* dextrose
- Dextrose 50% (unless patient is known to be euglycemic)
  - 50 mL IV in one dose
- Lorazepam (preferred initial benzodiazepine)
  - 0.05–0.1 mg/kg IV (range of 4–8 mg)
  - Do not exceed an infusion rate of 2 mg/min
  - Repeat every 5–15 min as needed up to three doses total
    - Maximum dosage equal to 8 mg
  - May administer IM in patients without IV access (maximum 3 mL per IM injection)
  - Patients on chronic benzodiazepine pharmacotherapy may require higher doses
- Diazepam
  - 0.1–0.3 mg/kg IV
  - Repeat every 10–20 min up to 30 mg total
  - Duration of effect is typically <20 min
  - May administer IM in patients without IV access (maximum 3 mL per IM injection)
- Phenytoin
  - 15–20 mg/kg IV
  - Do not exceed a rate of 50 mg/min
    - Do not exceed a rate of 25 mg/min in elderly patients or in the presence of atherosclerotic heart disease or conduction abnormalities
    - The infusion rate can be slowed if the seizure terminates or if an arrhythmia develops
  - If seizure persists, some experts administer an additional 5 mg/kg IV before advancing to the next line of pharmacotherapy
  - Target acute level 15–18 mcg/mL
    - Measure level 2 h after the initial loading dose
  - Equation to adjusted measured phenytoin levels in the setting of hypoalbuminemia
    - Adjusted phenytoin level equal to measured phenytoin level/(0.2 × serum albumin) + 0.1

- ○ Equation to adjust measured phenytoin levels in the setting of creatinine clearance ≤10 mL/min +/− hypoalbuminemia
  - ■ Adjusted phenytoin level = measured phenytoin level/(0.1 × serum albumin) + 0.1
- ○ Begin phenytoin maintenance dose 12 h after the loading dose if indicated
- Fosphenytoin (in place of phenytoin)
  - ○ 15–20 mg PE/kg IV
  - ○ Administered at a rate of 100–150 mg PE/min *(can give faster than phenytoin)*
  - ○ May administer IM in patients without IV access (maximum 3 mL per IM injection)
  - ○ If seizure persists, some experts administer an additional 5 mg PE/kg IV before advancing to the next line of pharmacotherapy
  - ○ Target acute phenytoin level 15–18 mcg/mL
    - ■ Measure level 2 h after the loading dose
  - ○ Begin *phenytoin* maintenance dose 12 h after the loading dose
- Phenobarbital
  - ○ 20 mg/kg IV
  - ○ Do not exceed a rate of 60–100 mg/min (ideal maximum is 60 mg/min)
    - ■ Use slower infusion rates in elderly patients
    - ■ The infusion rate can be slowed if the seizure terminates
  - ○ Target level 15–40 mcg/mL
  - ○ Give until seizure stops or until full dose administered
  - ○ May repeat 10–20 mg/kg IV if needed in 20 min
  - ○ May cause hypotension and respiratory depression
    - ■ Many experts would mechanically intubate the patient if a loading dose of phenobarbital is required

Refractory status epilepticus (patient must have a protected airway)
- Search for an acute or progressive etiology
- Midazolam
  - ○ 0.2 mg/kg IV, followed by 0.075–0.1 mg/kg/h continuous IV infusion

- ○ May administer IM in patients without IV access (maximum 3 mL per IM injection)
- ○ CYP450 enzyme induction from phenytoin, fosphenytoin, or barbiturates may decrease effect
- Propofol
  - ○ 1–2 mg/kg IV over 5 min, followed by 2–10 mg/kg/h continuous IV infusion
    - ▪ Reduce dose gradually 12 h after seizure cessation
  - ○ CYP450 enzyme induction from phenytoin, fosphenytoin, or barbiturates may decrease effect
- Pentobarbital
  - ○ 5 mg/kg IV over 1 h, followed by 0.5–3 mg/kg/h continuous IV infusion
  - ○ Administration rate should not exceed 50 mg/min
  - ○ Target level 20–40 mcg/mL
  - ○ Breakthrough seizure, 50 mg IV bolus, then increase the rate by 0.5–1 mg/kg/h
  - ○ Titrate to maintain burst suppression on electroencephalogram (EEG) or seizure cessation
    - ▪ 12 h after burst suppression, titrate downward every 4–6 h to evaluate remission
    - ▪ If breakthrough seizure, 50 mg IV bolus and increase infusion to closest preseizure dose
- Inhaled anesthetic agents in refractory cases
- Limited data on valproic acid
- Administer vitamin B_6 (pyridoxine) in the setting of isoniazid toxicity
  - ○ 1 g pyridoxine IV for each gram of isoniazid to a maximum of 5 g or 70 mg/kg
    - ▪ Repeat if necessary
  - ○ Alternative IV dosing regimen: 0.5 g/min until seizure stops or maximum dose is reached. When seizure stops, administer the remaining dose over 4–6 h

J. Neurol. 2003;250:401–406.
JAMA 1993;270:854–859.

Table 10.2
**Medications That May Exacerbate Weakness
in Myasthenia Gravis**

- Aminoglycosides, bacitracin, clindamycin, erythromycin, and polymixins
- Drugs with anticholinergic properties
  - Diphenhydramine, trihexiphenidyl, tricyclic antidepressants, phenothiazines, and lithium
- Procainamide, quinidine, quinine, disopyramide, phenytoin, and β-adrenergic blockers, calcium channel blockers
- Colchicine, cisplatinum, and penicillamine
- Magnesium-containing products (avoid hypermagnesemia)
- Neuromuscular blockers

Table 11.1
Nutrition Assessment

Body weight calculations
- Assess body mass index (weight in kg/height in m^2)
  - Underweight: <18.5
  - Normal weight: 18.5–24.9
  - Overweight: 25–29.9
  - Obese: 30–39.5
  - Extremely obese: ≥40
- Assess actual body weight (ABW)
  - Normal: 90–120% ideal body weight (IBW)
  - Mild malnutrition: 80–89% IBW
  - Moderate malnutrition: 70–79% IBW
  - Severe malnutrition: ≤69% IBW
  - Overweight: >120% IBW
  - Obese: ≥150% IBW
  - Extremely obese: ≥200% IBW
- IBW
  - Male = 50 kg + (2.3 × number of inches over 5 ft)
  - Female = 45.5 kg + (2.3 × number of inches over 5 ft)
- Adjusted nutrition body weight for overweight, obese, or extremely obese patients
  - Adjusted body weight = IBW + 0.3 (ABW – IBW)
  - Use this weight for nutritional calculations
- If ABW is less than IBW, use ABW

From: *Pocket Guide to Critical Care Pharmacotherapy*
By: J. Papadopoulos © Humana Press Inc., Totowa, NJ

Assessing daily caloric and protein needs
- Harris-Benedict equation to estimate caloric needs
  ○ Males
    ▪ (66 + 13.7 [wt in kg] + 5 [height in cm] – 6.8 [age]) ×
      AF × IF
  ○ Females
    ▪ (655 + 9.6 [wt in kg] + 1.8 [height in cm] – 4.7 [age]) ×
      AF × IF
  ○ Activity factors (AF)
    ▪ Out of bed: 1.3
    ▪ Fever: 1.13
  ○ Injury factors (IF)
    ▪ Infection: 1.2–1.8
    ▪ Surgery: 1.2–1.8
    ▪ Pancreatitis: 1–1.8
    ▪ Burns or head trauma: up to 2
- Protein needs assessment
  ○ Usual: 0.8 g/kg/d
  ○ Renal failure: <0.6 g/kg/d
  ○ Hemodialysis patients: 0.8–1.2 g/kg/d
  ○ CRRT: 1.2–1.5 g/kg/d
  ○ Liver failure: 0.5–1 g/kg/d
  ○ Critically ill patients: 1.2–2 g/kg/d
  ○ Burn patients: 2–3 g/kg/d
- Alternative to the Harris-Benedict equations
  ○ Maintenance or mild stress
    ▪ Total calories: 20–25 kcal/kg
    ▪ Nonprotein calories: 15–20 kcal/kg
    ▪ Daily protein needs: 0.5–1 g/kg
  ○ Mild-to-moderate stress (minor infection, disease
    exacerbation)
    ▪ Total calories: 25–30 kcal/kg
    ▪ Nonprotein calories: 20–25 kcal/kg
    ▪ Daily protein needs: 1–1.5 g/kg
  ○ Moderate-to-severe stress (sepsis, major surgery, and burns)
    ▪ Total calories: 30–35 kcal/kg

- Nonprotein calories: 25–30 kcal/kg
  - Daily protein needs: 1.5–2 g/kg (>2 g/kg for burn patients ≥30% body surface area)
- Nonprotein calorie to nitrogen ratio (NPC/N)
  - Nitrogen = grams of protein/6.25
  - Maintenance NPC/N ratio: 150:1
  - Stress NPC/N ratio: 90–120:1

Macronutrients
- Carbohydrates
  - Provides 3.4 kcal/g parenterally and 4 kcal/g enterally
  - Should not exceed 5 mg/kg/min parenterally. Can result in:
    - Increased carbon dioxide production
    - Hyperglycemia
    - Lipogenesis
    - Cholestasis (increased total bilirubin, direct bilirubin, alkaline phosphatase, and γ-glutamyl transferase)
- Lipids
  - Provides 10 kcal/g
  - Do not exceed 1 g/kg/d or 60% of total calories
  - Do not administer in patients with egg allergies
  - Adverse effects include
    - Dyspnea, chest pain, palpitations, and chills
    - Headaches, nausea, and fever
    - Cholestasis (increased total bilirubin, direct bilirubin, alkaline phosphatase, and γ-glutamyl transferase)
- Protein
  - Provides 4 kcal/g
  - In critically ill patients, may give protein calories in excess of energy requirements in order for this macronutrient to be utilized for tissue repair and synthesis (controversial)
    - i.e., give total calories as nonprotein calories

CRRT, continuous renal replacement techniques.

Table 11.2
Principles of Parenteral Nutrition (Consult a Nutrition Expert Wherever Appropriate)

Indications
- Inability to absorb nutrients from the gastrointestinal tract
  - Small bowel resection, severe diarrhea, intractable vomiting, bowel obstruction, and fistulas
  - Critically ill patients with nonfunctioning GI tract
    - Sepsis, trauma, cancer, and severe pancreatitis
- Hyperemesis gravidarum
- Severe malnutrition

Routes
- Peripheral vein
  - Used in patients without large nutritional requirements and fluid not restricted
  - Cannot exceed 850–900 mOsm/L solutions
    - Amino acids provide 10 mOsm/g
    - Dextrose provides 5 mOsm/g
    - Lipids provides 0.71 mOsm/g (product specific)
  - Complications include thrombophlebitis
- Central vein
  - Patients who require parenteral nutrition for >7 d
  - Must be administered through a central vein
    - Subclavian and internal jugular
  - Must verify catheter placement

Initiating
- Determine caloric needs (refer to Table 11.1)
  - 50% estimated caloric needs first day
  - 75–100% estimated caloric needs by second to third day
- Determine protein needs
- Determine route

- Titrate macronutrients based on
  - Substrate tolerance
  - Patient's body weight
  - Biochemical markers (e.g., prealbumin)
  - 24-h urine urea nitrogen collection in critically ill patients

Discontinuing
- When discontinuing parenteral nutrition, it is important to taper over several days to prevent hypoglycemia
- If parenteral nutrition is stopped abruptly, replace with a dextrose 10% in water solution and infuse at the same parenteral nutrition rate

---

Table 11.3
Select Drug–Nutrient Interactions

- Phenytoin
  - Caseinate salts found in enteral nutrition formulas may reduce bioavailability (mechanism not well delineated)
  - Protocol
    - Hold feeds 1–2 h before and after administration
    - Flush enteral feeding tube with 20 mL water or saline
    - Administer dose
    - Adjust enteral feeding rate to maintain the same 24-h volume
- Warfarin
  - Vitamin K content of enteral nutrition formulas may affect pharmacological activity. Monitor and titrate dose to maintain therapeutic international normalized ratio (INR)
- Medications with a decreased bioavailability if administered concomitantly with enteral nutrition formulas
  - Azithromycin, fluoroquinolones, ketoconazole, isoniazid, penicillin, rifampin, and tetracycline
  - Didanosine, indinavir, stavudine, and zidovudine
  - Aledronate, risedronate, and levodopa

Table 11.4
Strategies to Minimize Aspiration of Gastric Contents during Enteral Nutrition

- Start desired enteral nutrition product at 20 mL/h
  - Increase every 6 h by 20 mL/h increments until goal rate achieved
- Check gastric residuals every 8–12 h
  - Keep ≤150 mL
- Use continuous infusion instead of intermittent bolus feeding
- Elevate head of bed by a 30–45° angle
- Consider continuous subglottic suctioning in mechanically ventilated patients
- Optimizing oral health
- The use of blue food coloring and methylene blue should be avoided, as it has low sensitivity and has been associated with adverse patient outcomes

If high gastric residuals
- Prokinetic agents
  - Metoclopramide
    - 5–10 mg IV every 6–8 h (adjust for renal impairment)
  - Erythromycin
    - 250 mg IV or enterally every 6–8 h for ≤5 d
- Minimize use of narcotic analgesics wherever possible
  - Enteral naloxone (parenteral product)
    - 1–2 mg *enterally* every 6 h may decrease the gastrointestinal effect of opioid analgesics without reversing the systemic analgesic effects. Monitor for opioid withdrawal
- Transpyloric or small bowel feeding
  - Positioning the tip of the feeding tube past the ligament of Treitz may be more effective than postpyloric placement in high-risk patients

Chest 2004;125:793–795.
JPEN 2002;26:S80–S85.

Psychiatric Disorders

Table 12.1
Management of Alcohol Withdrawal

Refer to the clinical institute withdrawal assessment for alcohol scale (CIWA-Ar)
- A validated 10-item assessment tool used to monitor the severity of withdrawal and monitor pharmacotherapy
  - A score of ≤8 corresponds to mild withdrawal
  - A score between 9 and 15 corresponds to moderate withdrawal
  - A score of more than 15 corresponds to severe withdrawal and at increased risk of seizures and delirium tremens

Supportive care
- Intravenous fluids
- Correct any electrolyte abnormalities
- Thiamine 100 mg IV/enterally daily
  - Administer before glucose administration to prevent precipitation of Wernicke's encephalopathy
- Multivitamin daily (source of folate)
- Avoid phenothiazines and haloperidol, as both may lower the seizure threshold

Benzodiazepine pharmacotherapy
- Fixed dose regimens
  - Administered at specific intervals with additional doses given as needed

From: *Pocket Guide to Critical Care Pharmacotherapy*
By: J. Papadopoulos © Humana Press Inc., Totowa, NJ

- ○ Chlordiazepoxide 50–100 mg enterally every 6 h for 1 d, 25–50 mg every 6 h for 2 d then continue to taper for a total of 7 d
- ○ In patients with significant liver dysfunction, lorazepam or oxazepam may be preferred
- ○ This regimen is useful in patients at high risk of major withdrawal or history of withdrawal seizures or delirium tremens
- Loading dose strategy
  - ○ Diazepam 10–20 mg enterally initially to provide sedation
  - ○ Titrate additional doses every 5–15 min until goal achieved
  - ○ Then allow the drug level to taper through metabolism
- Symptom-triggered regimens
  - ○ Administered only when the CIWA-Ar score is ≥9. May administer with a lower threshold (i.e., CIWA-Ar score <9) if there is a history of withdrawal seizures
    - ■ Administer diazepam 5 mg IV/enterally initially. Measure the CIWA-Ar score 1 h after the initial and each subsequent dose of diazepam. Adjust dose based on severity of symptoms
    - ■ Alternative may be chlordiazepoxide 25–50 mg IV/enterally every hour as needed
  - ○ This approach may result in less total medication and more rapid detoxification

Other pharmacotherapy for alcohol withdrawal symptoms
- Phenobarbital
- Carbamazepine
- Ethanol (enteral and parenteral)

Adjuvant pharmacotherapy
- Sympatholytics
  - ○ β-adrenergic blockers or clonidine may be utilized in conjunction with benzodiazepines in patients with coronary artery disease who may not tolerate adrenergic excess
  - ○ Limited experience with dexmedetomidine
- Benzodiazepine refractory delirium tremens
  - ○ Consider propofol pharmacotherapy, as it agonizes GABA-A receptors and antagonizes NMDA receptors. Phenobarbital can be used as an alternative

*Anticonvulsant pharmacotherapy for status epilepticus
(uncommon—consider alternative etiology)*
- Low threshold for airway protection and mechanical ventilation
- Benzodiazepines
- Phenytoin
- Propofol

CIWA-Ar, Clinical Institute Withdrawal Assessment for Alcohol-Revised;
GABA, γ-aminobutyric acid; IV, intravenous; NMDA, *N*-methyl *D*-aspartate.
Br. J. Addict. 1989;84:1353–1357.
Am. Fam. Physician 2004;69:1443–1450.
NEJM 2003;348:1786–1795.
Crit. Care Med. 2000;28:1781–1784.

Table 12.2
Management of Serotonin Syndrome

*Precipitating medications (usually when utilized in combination
or inadequate washout period)*
- Serotonin reuptake inhibitors
  - Citalopram, escitalopram, fluoxetine, fluvoxamine, paroxetine,
    and sertraline
  - Clomipramine, imipramine, nefazodone, trazodone, and
    venlafaxine
  - Dextromethorphan, meperidine, and pentazocine
  - Amphetamine, fenfluoramine, dexfenfluoramine,
    methylphenidate, and cocaine
  - Sibutramine, St. John's wort, ondansetron, granisetron,
    dolasetron, and palonosetron
- Enhance serotonin release
  - Methylenedioxymethamphetamine (MDMA or ecstasy)
    or mirtazapine
- Serotonin receptor agonists
  - Buspirone, lithium, and ergot alkaloids
  - Lysergic acid diethylamide (LSD)
- Serotonin precursor
  - L-tryptophan
- Impair serotonin breakdown
  - Monamine oxidase inhibitors
    - Isocarboxizid, phenelzine, selegiline, tranylcypromine,
      moclobemide, clorgiline, and linezolid

Signs and symptoms
- Typically start within minutes to hours after ingestion
- Usually resolve within 12–24 h with cessation of precipitating agent or supportive therapy but can be prolonged with long half-life drugs
- Assess for the presence of the following clinical features
  - Agitation, altered mental status, delirium, diaphoresis, diarrhea, and hyperactive bowel sounds
  - Hyperreflexia (L > U extremities), hyperthermia, and incoordination
    - Poorly treated hyperthermia may lead to metabolic acidosis, rhabdomyolysis, elevated aminotransferases, seizures, renal failure, and disseminated intravascular coagulation (DIC)
  - Myoclonus (inducible or spontaneous), muscular hypertonicity, shivering, tremor, akathesia, tachycardia, mydriasis, and ocular clonus
  - Severe symptomatology may mask other clinical features

Management depends on the severity of illness
- Discontinue offending agent(s)
- Supportive care
  - Fluids to replace hyperthermia-induced and gastrointestinal losses
  - Hemodynamic support if necessary
- Rapid external cooling for hyperthermic patients
  - Fans, cooling blankets, and tepid water baths. For severe cases consider sedation and neuromuscular paralysis. No role for antipyretic pharmacotherapy
- Intravenous benzodiazepine to decrease muscle rigidity and agitation
- Cyproheptadine
  - *Mild-to-moderate cases:* 4 mg enterally q8h
  - *Severe cases:* 12 mg enterally in one dose, then 2 mg every 2 h as symptoms continue. Once signs and symptoms are controlled, convert to 8 mg enterally every 6 h
  - Duration patient and agent specific

- Avoid
  - Physical restraints (may be associated with isometric muscle contractions and worsening of hyperthermia)
  - Propranolol (may worsen autonomic instability)

NEJM 2005;352:1112–1120.
Am. J. Resp. Crit. Care Med. 2002;166:9–15.
Ann. Emerg. Med. 1996;28:520–526.
Am. J. Psychiatry 1991;148:705–713.

Table 12.3
Management of Neuroleptic Malignant Syndrome

Precipitating medications
- Typical and atypical antipsychotic medications (D_2-receptor antagonists)
  - Haloperidol, phenothiazines, thioxanthenes, clozapine, olanzapine, quetiapine, and risperidone
  - Parenteral agents may have a higher incidence
- Droperidol, metoclopramide, prochlorperazine, promethazine, venlafaxine, and reserpine
- Abrupt withdrawal of dopamine agonists
  - Levodopa, bromocriptine, and amantadine

Signs and symptoms
- Altered consciousness
- Autonomic instability (e.g., labile blood pressure, tachycardia, diaphoresis, and incontinence)
- Hyperthermia
- Rigidity (lead-pipe)
- May occur within the first few weeks of pharmacotherapy or with rapid increases in dose
- Once neuroleptic malignant syndrome (NMS) develops, signs and symptoms may escalate over 24–72 h and may have a prolonged clinical course

Management
- Discontinue offending agent

- Rapid external cooling
  - Fans, cooling blankets, and tepid water baths
  - Consider core cooling in acute severe hyperthermia
  - Antipyretic pharmacotherapy is not effective
- Fluids
  - To replace hyperthermia-induced losses
- Intravenous benzodiazepine to decrease muscle rigidity
- Bromocriptine 2.5–5 mg enterally tid (can be increased to 30–45 mg/d)
- Dantrolene IV
  - 2.5 mg/kg IV every 5–10 min as necessary up to a maximum of 10 mg/kg
  - Then, 1–2 mg/kg enterally q6h for 72 h
  - Role not well delineated in NMS
- Other interventions
  - Restart medication (e.g., levodopa) if episode is believed to be a result of drug withdrawal
  - Anticholinergic agents should not be abruptly withdrawn but use may be a confounding variable in the setting of hyperthermia
  - Electroconvulsive therapy may be useful in drug-refractory cases
  - Nondepolarizing neuromuscular blockers may be useful in severe, refractory cases
  - If antipsychotic pharmacotherapy is still warranted
    - Wait until 1–2 wk after symptoms have resolved
    - Initiate therapy with an agent from a different class
    - Select a low-potency or atypical agent and adjust therapy using the lowest possible dose

Psychiatric Quarterly 2001;72:325–336.

Table 13.1
Management of Chronic Obstructive Pulmonary Disease

Management of stable disease
- Stage 0—at risk
  - Normal spirometry
  - Avoidance of risk factors
  - Influenza vaccine
- Stage I—mild disease
  - $FEV_1/FVC < 70\%$
  - $FEV_1 \geq 80\%$
  - Add short-acting bronchodilator (i.e., albuterol prn and ipratropium)
- Stage II—moderate disease
  - $FEV_1/FVC < 70\%$
  - $FEV_1 < 80\%$ and $\geq 50\%$
  - Add short-acting bronchodilator (i.e., albuterol prn and ipratropium)
  - Add standing treatment with one or more long-acting bronchodilators (i.e., tiotropium, salmeterol, and formoterol)
  - Add rehabilitation
- Stage III—severe disease
  - $FEV_1/FVC < 70\%$
  - $FEV_1 < 50\%$ and $\geq 30\%$
  - Add short-acting bronchodilator (i.e., albuterol prn and ipratropium)

From: *Pocket Guide to Critical Care Pharmacotherapy*
By: J. Papadopoulos © Humana Press Inc., Totowa, NJ

- ○ Add standing treatment with one or more long-acting bronchodilators (i.e., tiotropium, salmeterol, and formoterol)
- ○ Add inhaled corticosteroid therapy if repeat exacerbations
  - ▪ Discontinue if no clinical or spirometric response
- ○ Add rehabilitation
- Stage IV—very severe disease
  - ○ $FEV_1/FVC < 70\%$
  - ○ $FEV_1 < 30\%$ or presence of chronic respiratory failure or right heart failure
  - ○ Add short-acting bronchodilator (i.e., albuterol prn and ipratropium)
  - ○ Add standing treatment with one or more long-acting bronchodilators (i.e., tiotropium, salmeterol, and formoterol)
  - ○ Add inhaled corticosteroid therapy if repeat exacerbations
    - ▪ Discontinue if no clinical or spirometric response
  - ○ Add rehabilitation
  - ○ Add long-term oxygen therapy if chronic respiratory failure
  - ○ Consider surgical treatments

In-patient management of acute exacerbations
- Oxygen therapy
- Nebulized short-acting bronchodilator therapy (e.g., albuterol and ipratropium)
- Consider intravenous aminophylline if needed
- Corticosteroid therapy
  - ○ Prednisone 40 mg enterally daily or equivalent for 10–14 d
- Antimicrobials therapy if increased sputum volume or change in color
  - ○ Cover *Streptococcus pneumoniae, Hemophilus influenza, Moraxella catarrhalis*
  - ○ Evaluate antimicrobial use in the past 3 mo to determine possible pathogen and optimal antimicrobial agent

www.goldcopd.com.

Table 13.2
Management of Acute Asthma Exacerbations

Initial therapy
- Albuterol
  - 2.5–5 mg nebulized every 20 min for 1 h or 10–15 mg/h continuously for 1 h
    - Driven by oxygen instead of air
    - A metered dose inhaler with spacer is equivalent to nebulized therapy, may have a more rapid onset, and fewer adverse effects
      - 4–8 puff doses
- Oxygen to achieve an oxygen saturation ≥90%
- Systemic corticosteroids if no immediate response or incomplete response to aggressive inhaled β_2-adrenergic agonist therapy, if patient recently received an oral corticosteroid, or if the episode is considered severe
  - Prednisone or methylprednisolone 60–80 mg/d or equivalent in three to four divided doses for 48 h, then 30–40 mg/d or equivalent in two divided doses until PEF ≥80% personal best
    - Usually a 7–14 d course is adequate
  - No proven benefit of intravenous over oral therapy
  - No proven benefit of tapering dose
- Avoid drugs that cause histamine release (e.g., morphine sulfate, codeine, atracurium, metocurine, mivacurium, and tubocurarine)

Assessment after initial therapy
- Moderate episode (PEF 60–80% predicted/personal best, moderate symptoms, accessory muscle use)
  - Albuterol 2.5–5 mg nebulized every hour
  - Ipratropium 500 mcg nebulized every hour
  - Continue therapy for 1–3 h, provided there is improvement
  - Consider corticosteroid
    - Prednisone or methylprednisolone 60–80 mg/d or equivalent in three to four divided doses
- Severe episode (PEF < 60% predicted/personal best, severe symptoms at rest, and chest retraction)
  - Albuterol 2.5–5 mg nebulized every hour
  - Ipratropium 500 mcg nebulized every hour

- ○ Oxygen therapy
- ○ Systemic corticosteroid (intravenous)
- ○ Consider systemic β_2-adrenergic agonist
  - Epinephrine (1:1000)
  - 0.3–0.5 mg (0.3–0.5 mL of the 1:1000 solution) SQ every 20 min for three doses
  - Terbutaline
  - 0.25 mg SQ every 15–30 min for two doses
  - Consider intravenous aminophylline
  - Target theophylline level between 5 and 15 mcg/mL
  - Consider magnesium 2 g intravenously for over 20 min
- ○ If sedation is required, consider either propofol (preferred) or ketamine, as both drugs are weak bronchodilators
- • Notes
  - ○ The dose-response curve for β_2-adrenergic agonists is shifted to the right with increased levels of bronchoconstriction. This explains the need for higher and more frequent doses during an acute asthma exacerbation
  - ○ The dose of bronchodilator can be gradually reduced based on both symptomatic and objective improvement until the patient returns to pre-exacerbation use of short-acting β_2-adrenergic agonist pharmacotherapy
  - ○ Discontinue ipratropium pharmacotherapy after the acute phase of treatment, as it is unlikely that it will provide any additional benefit
  - ○ Discontinue long-acting β_2-adrenergic agonist therapy during the acute phase of treatment
  - ○ Levalbuterol may be utilized if the patient experiences tachycardia or tremors with albuterol
  - ○ Antimicrobials should be reserved for patients with evidence of a bacterial respiratory tract infection

Response in E.R. and placement
- • Good response
  - ○ Sustained 60 min after last treatment
  - ○ Normal physical examination and no distress
  - ○ PEF > 70%

- ○ Oxygen saturation > 90%
- ○ Discharge home
  - ■ Adjust pharmacotherapy
  - ■ Consider in most cases a short-course of an oral corticosteroid
  - ■ Review peak flow meter and inhaler technique
  - ■ Identify precipitating factors
  - ■ Recommend close medical follow-up
- Incomplete response after 1–2 h
  - ○ Mild-to-moderate symptoms on physical exam
  - ○ PEF < 70%
  - ○ Oxygen saturation not improving
  - ○ Admit to hospital ward
    - ■ Inhaled albuterol +/– ipratropium pharmacotherapy
    - ■ Systemic corticosteroid (oral or intravenous)
    - ■ Oxygen therapy
    - ■ Consider intravenous aminophylline
  - ○ Can discharge home if PEF > 60% predicted/personal best and sustained on inhaled/oral therapy
    - ■ Adjust pharmacotherapy
    - ■ Continue a short-course of an oral corticosteroid
    - ■ Review peak flow meter and inhaler technique
    - ■ Identify precipitating factors
    - ■ Recommend close medical follow-up
  - ○ If no improvement, admit into an intensive care unit
- Poor response within 1 h
  - ○ Severe symptoms, altered level of consciousness
  - ○ PEF < 30%
  - ○ $PaCO_2 > 45$
  - ○ $PaO_2 < 60$
  - ○ Admit to an intensive care unit
    - ■ Inhaled albuterol and ipratropium pharmacotherapy
    - ■ Systemic corticosteroid (intravenous)
    - ■ Oxygen therapy
    - ■ Consider systemic β_2-adrenergic agonist pharmacotherapy
    - ■ Consider intravenous aminophylline
    - ■ Possible intubation and mechanical ventilation

Triggers
- Acute exacerbations usually result from an allergen or a viral infection
- Gradual exacerbations may reflect failure of long-term pharmacotherapy
- For a complete list of triggers, refer to the aforementioned internet address

www.ginasthma.com.

Table 13.3
Drug-Induced Pulmonary Diseases

Cough
- Angiotensin converting enzyme inhibitors

Eosinophilic pulmonary infiltration
- Nitrofurantoin, penicillin, and sulfonamide antimicrobials
- Aspirin and NSAIDs
- Amiodarone, bleomycin, captopril, chlorpropamide, chlorpromazine, imipramine, methotrexate, and phenytoin

Noncardiogenic (permeability) pulmonary edema
- Morphine, heroin, methadone, and propoxyphene
- Naloxone and nalmefene
- Salicylates and hydrochlorothiazide
- Bleomycin, cyclophosphamide, mitomycin, vinblastine, and interleukin-2

Pneumonitis
- Amiodarone, docetaxel, gold compounds, and nitrofurantoin, paclitaxel

Pulmonary fibrosis
- Bleomycin, busulfan, carmustine, cyclophosphamide, methotrexate, mitomycin, and radiation therapy
- Amiodarone, methysergide, and nitrofurantoin

Table 14.1
Contrast-Induced Nephropathy Prevention Strategy[a]

Risk factors
- Creatinine clearance < 60 mL/min/1.73 m² (stages III–V chronic kidney disease), diabetes mellitus (with renal insufficiency), hypertension, chronic heart failure, cirrhosis, nephrosis, age >75 yr, cholesterol emboli syndrome, multiple myeloma (questionable)
- Hypovolemia, intraprocedural volume depletion, use of large volumes of contrast, and intra-aortic balloon pump
- Urine albumin/creatinine ratio >30, proteinuria
- Concurrent nephrotoxin use (e.g., aminoglycosides, polymixins, amphotericin B, foscarnet, cyclosporine, tacrolimus, and NSAIDs)
- Other medications (e.g., angiotensin converting enzyme inhibitors, angiotensin receptor blockers, and diuretics)
- Intra-arterial contrast administration may have a higher prevalence than the intravenous route

The first preventative strategy is to address any reversible risk factor(s)[b]

Hydration with normal saline or sodium bicarbonate (3 amps NaHCO₃/1L D5W) solutions
- Use if there are no contraindications to volume expansion
- Hold diuretics day before and of procedure
- Isotonic saline preferred over 0.45% saline
  - Start 2 h (up to 12 h in high-risk patients) before procedure
    - 1 mL/kg/h

From: *Pocket Guide to Critical Care Pharmacotherapy*
By: J. Papadopoulos © Humana Press Inc., Totowa, NJ

○ Continue for at least 6 h after the procedure
○ Target urine output around 150 mL/h
- Sodium bicarbonate found to be more effective than isotonic saline hydration.[c] Some clinicians have questioned this trial's methodology
  ○ 3 mL/kg/h for 1 h before contrast
  ○ 1 mL/kg/h for 6 h after procedure

Contrast agent
- Use nonionic and either low or iso-osmolal products
  ○ Example, iodixanol
- Use least amount of volume to complete the procedure
  ○ A volume >5 mL/kg divided by serum creatinine in mg/dL associated with increased risk of nephropathy
- Avoid studies that are closely spaced. Optimal time not well delineated. Prudent to wait a few days between studies when possible

Pharmacotherapy
- N-acetylcysteine (NAC)
  ○ Enterally 600 mg q12h (24 h before and 24 h after the procedure)
    ▪ For emergent procedures, 1 g of NAC for 1 h before and 4 h after the procedure may have some value[d]
  ○ Intravenous
    ▪ 150 mg/kg in 500 mL normal saline over 30 min before procedure, followed by 50 mg/kg in 500 mL normal saline over 4 h following the procedure[e]

Limited if any value based on the available literature
- Forced diuresis with either a loop diuretic or mannitol
- Renal dose dopamine
- Aminophylline/theophylline (adenosine receptor antagonists)
- Calcium-channel blockers
- Fenoldopam
- Hemodialysis or hemofiltration

---

[a]*NEJM* 2006;354:379–386; *Crit. Care Clin.* 2005;21:261–280.
[b]A risk prediction table can be found in *NEJM 2006;354:379–386.*
[c]*JAMA* 2004;291:2328–2334.
[d]*J. Interv. Cardiol.* 2004;17(3):159–165.
[e]*J. Am. Coll. Cardiol.* 2003;41(12):2114–2118.

Table 14.2
Pharmacological Management of Acute Renal Failure

Fluid control (must assess patient's volume status)
- Intravascular deplete
  - Administer crystalloid fluid resuscitation
- Volume overloaded
  - Concentrate intravenous medications
  - Evaluate maintenance fluids
  - Concentrate parenteral nutrition
  - Use concentrated enteral nutrition products

Avoid and/or discontinue nephrotoxins wherever possible

Diuretic pharmacotherapy (strict avoidance of intravascular volume depletion)
- Loop diuretics *(dose depends on severity of renal insufficiency)*
  - Not directly beneficial in established acute tubular necrosis. Animal studies suggest benefit but human trials are conflicting. More studies are needed.
  - Furosemide intermittent IV
    - Rate ≤4 mg/min for doses ≥100 mg
    - 40–80 mg intravenous push (IVP)
      - If net hourly diuresis is >1 mL/kg/h and pharmacotherapeutic end point is achieved, then no further diuretic
      - If net hourly diuresis is ≥1 mL/kg/h and pharmacotherapeutic end point is not achieved, then continue same dose every 6 h
      - If net hourly diuresis is <1 mL/kg/h, double the previous dose of diuretic and administer within 2 h
        - Consider combining with a thiazide diuretic
  - Furosemide continuous IV infusion
    - 40–100 mg intravenous bolus
    - Initiate at 0.1 mg/kg/h continuous IV infusion
      - Increase hourly by 0.1 mg/kg/h increments until net hourly diuresis is ≥1 mL/kg/h
      - Maximum rate is 0.4–0.5 mg/kg/h
      - Continue until pharmacotherapeutic end point is achieved
        - Consider combining with a thiazide diuretic if large doses of furosemide are required

- Thiazide diuretics
  - May have synergistic activity with a loop diuretic
  - Chlorothiazide
    - 500–1000 mg IV q12h
    - Avoid or use cautiously if patient's estimated creatinine clearance is <20 mL/min
  - Metolazone
    - 5–20 mg enterally daily
    - Unlike thiazide diuretics, may produce effective diuresis at creatinine clearances <20 mL/min
- In "sulfa" allergic patients:
  - Identify the implicated agent and the severity of reaction
  - Ethacrynic acid may be a safe alternative to furosemide
    - 40 mg furosemide = 50 mg ethacrynic acid
  - Refer to the following review article on sulfonamide allergies[a]

Management of diuretic-resistant edema
- Evaluate excessive sodium intake
  - Dietary, intravenous fluids, medications (e.g., ticarcillin, metronidazole)
- Switch to parenteral diuretic pharmacotherapy
- Increase dose of loop diuretic
- Consider continuous infusion of a loop diuretic
- Consider combining the loop diuretic with either a thiazide diuretic or metolazone
- Discontinue medications that may decrease renal blood flow
  - E.g., angiotensin converting enzyme inhibitors, angiotensin receptor blockers, and NSAIDs
- Combined loop diuretic and albumin
  - Data supporting efficacy is limited
  - Albumin 12.5–25 g IV every 8–24 h
  - Use only if diuretics have been maximized
  - May be warranted in patients with severe hypoalbuminemia

---

[a]*Ann. Pharmacother.* 2005;39:290–301.

Table 14.3
Management of Acute Uremic Bleeding

- Packed red blood cell transfusion (PRBCs)
  - Goal hematocrit ≥28 – 30% (patient specific)
  - Higher hematocrit may improve platelet-vessel wall interaction
- Cryoprecipitate (in life-threatening hemorrhage)
  - 10 units every 12–24 h
  - To replenish von Willebrand factor (vWF)
- Desmopressin
  - 0.3 mcg/kg IV over 15 -30 min
  - May repeat q12h for 2–3 total doses
    - Will increase endothelial release of vWF
    - Tachyphylaxis develops with repeat doses. Activity may return after a 3-d drug-free period
- Conjugated estrogen in severe cases
  - 0.6 mg/kg IV daily for 5 d

Table 14.4
Drug-Induced Renal Disease

Functional acute renal failure
- Angiotensin converting enzyme inhibitors, angiotensin receptor blockers, and NSAIDs

Glomerular disease
- Gold, hydralazine, and NSAIDs
- Chlorpropamide, penicillamine, phenytoin, and quinidine

Interstitial nephritis
- Acute allergic
  - β-lactam antimicrobials, erythromycin, nitrofurantoin, rifampin, sulfonamide antimicrobials, and vancomycin
  - Diuretics (all classes), NSAIDs
- Chronic
  - Cyclosporine, ifosfamide, and lithium

Obstructive nephropathy
- Intratubular
  - Acyclovir, foscarnet, indinavir, and sulfonamide antimicrobials
  - Acetazolamide, ascorbic acid, methotrexate, and triamterene
- Outflow obstruction
  - Anticholinergic agents and disopyramide
- Nephrolithiasis
  - Allopurinol, indinavir, sulfadiazine, topiramate, triamterene, and zonisamide
- Rhabdomyolysis
  - Azathioprine, colchicine, niacin (in combination with a statin), and statins

Papillary necrosis
- Acetaminophen

Pseudorenal failure (increase in blood urea nitrogen or serum creatinine without a change in glomerular filtration rate)
- Increase protein catabolism
  - Corticosteroids and tetracyclines
- Impairs proximal tubular secretion of creatinine
  - Cimetidine, pyrimethamine, and trimethoprim
- Interactions with laboratory assay (Jaffe method)
  - Ascorbic acid
  - Cephalosporins (e.g., cefazolin, cefoxitin, cefaclor, cephalexin, and cephalothin)

Tubular damage
- Acute tubular necrosis
  - Aminoglycosides, amphotericin B, carboplatin, cisplatin, foscarnet, and intravenous contrast dyes
- Osmotic damage
  - Dextrans, mannitol, intravenous immunoglobulin, and hetastarch

Table 14.5
Management of Acute Hypocalcemia
(Serum Calcium <8.5 mg/dL)

- Correct serum calcium in the presence of hypoalbuminemia
  - Corrected serum calcium (mg/dL) = measured serum calcium (mg/dL) + 0.8 (4 g/dL – measured serum albumin [g/dL])
  - Measure ionized calcium levels (normal 4–5.2 mg/dL or 1–1.3 mmol/L)
    - Preferred approach in critically-ill patients
- Evaluate and manage etiology
  - Check parathyroid hormone (PTH), vitamin D and precursors, magnesium, and phosphate levels
  - Pharmacological causes of decreased ionized calcium may include excess infusions of citrate, EDTA, lactate, fluoride poisoning, foscarnet, cinacalcet, bisphosphates, or unrelated increase in serum phosphate or decrease in serum magnesium levels
- Symptomatic (e.g., dysrhythmias, hypotension, tetany, and seizures)
  - Calcium chloride 1 g (10 mL of a 10% solution) IV over 5–10 min
    - Usually associated with an ionized calcium level of <2.8 mg/dL or 0.7 mmol/L
    - Contains 272 mg/13.6 mEq elemental calcium per gram product
    - Severe desiccant → give through a central line
  - Calcium gluconate 1–3 g (10–30 mL of a 10% solution) IV over 5–10 min
    - Contains 93 mg/4.5 mEq elemental calcium per gram product
    - Preferred product for peripheral venous administration
  - Measure serum calcium every 6 h during acute therapy
  - A continuous IV infusion of 0.3–2 mg/kg/h may be initiated to achieve and maintain normocalcemia

- ○ Change to enteral therapy once serum calcium is ≥8.5 mg/dL or ionized calcium normalizes
- ○ Use cautiously in patients on digitalis glycoside pharmacotherapy
- ○ Correct concomitant hypomagnesemia
- ○ Initiate calcitriol 0.25 mcg enterally daily if suspect vitamin D or PTH deficiency
  - ▪ Switch to nonhydroxylated form after 1 wk in patients without renal failure, PTH resistance, or PTH failure
- ○ If present and clinically feasible, treat acute severe hyper-phosphatemia before calcium administration (i.e., with hemodialysis in acute tumor lysis syndrome)
- • Asymptomatic
  - ○ Enteral calcium 1–3 g daily
  - ○ Various salts
    - ▪ Carbonate: 250 mg elemental calcium per 500 mg tablet
    - ▪ Citrate: 200 mg elemental calcium per 950 mg tablet
    - ▪ Gluconate: 90 mg elemental calcium per 1 g tablet
    - ▪ Lactate: 60 mg elemental calcium per 300 mg tablet
  - ○ Calcium citrate and gluconate do not require an acidic medium for maximal bioavailability (i.e., appropriate salt for concomitant acid suppressive therapy)

Table 14.6
Management of Acute Hypercalcemia
(Serum Calcium >12 mg/dL)

- • Identify and manage etiology (e.g., hyperparathyroidism, malignancy)
  - ○ Drug-induced causes can include:
    - ▪ Thiazide diuretics, calcium-containing antacids, vitamin D, and lithium
- • Intravenous 0.9% saline (if no contraindications are present)
  - ○ 200–300 mL/h initial therapy (patient-specific)
  - ○ 100–200 mL/h once patient is adequately hydrated
  - ○ Maintain urine output between 100 and 150 mL/h

- Potassium and magnesium supplementation
- Loop diuretics
  - Patient must be adequately rehydrated before use
    - May worsen hypercalcemia in hypovolemic patients by promoting tubular calcium reabsorption
  - Example, furosemide 40–80 mg IV (1 mg/kg) every 2–4 h
- Calcitonin salmon four units/kg SQ q12h
  - Onset within 1–2 h
  - A test dose should be considered before therapy is initiated
    - In a tuberculin syringe dilute 10 units in 1 mL 0.9% saline
    - Inject one unit (0.1 mL) intradermally on the flexor surface of the forearm
      - □ The appearance of erythema or a wheal within 15 min indicates a positive reaction, and calcitonin salmon should not be administered
  - If an inadequate response is observed after 1–2 d, may increase the dose to eight units/kg SQ every 12 h
  - Tachyphylaxis may develop (limit use to 48 h)
- Bisphosphonate
  - Slow onset (1–2 d)
  - Use cautiously in patients with renal insufficiency
  - Etidronate 7.5 mg/kg IV over 2–4 h for 3–5 d
  - Pamidronate 60–90 mg IV × 1 dose over 2 h
    - 60 mg for calcium levels ≤13.5 mg/dL
    - 90 mg for calcium levels >13.5 mg/dL
  - Zoledronate 4 mg IV in one dose over 15 min (preferred agent)
- Other agents
  - Gallium nitrate 200 mg/m^2/d by continuous IV infusion for ≤5 d
    - May be superior to bisphosphonates for humoral hyper-calcemia of malignancy (PTHrp)
  - Glucocorticoids
    - Prednisone 20–40 mg enterally daily or equivalent if lymphoma or granulomatous disease-related
  - Chelating agents (rarely used)
    - EDTA 10–50 mg/kg over 4 h up to a maximum of 3 g in 24 h

- Hemodialysis with calcium-free dialysate
  - In life-threatening situations or if the patient is anuric

---

Table 14.7
Management of Acute Hypokalemia
(Serum Potassium <3.5 mEq/L)

- Evaluate etiology
  - Drug-induced may include:
    - Diuretics, and laxatives
    - Sympathomimetics (including inhaled/nebulized B_2-adrenergic agonists), theophylline, and caffeine
    - Penicillin, ampicillin, nafcillin, ticarcillin, aminoglycosides, and amphotericin B
    - Cisplatin
- Symptomatic or severe hypokalemia (<2.5 mEq/L)
  - 10–20 mEq over 1 h
  - Repeat as necessary until serum potassium normalizes
  - Electrocardiogram monitoring is indicated when infusion rates exceed 10 mEq/h
  - Doses >20 mEq/h should be administered through a central line
    - Catheter tip should not be extended into the right atrium
  - Maximum rate is 40 mEq/h
  - Parenteral product should be mixed with saline instead of dextrose diluents
    - To prevent insulin-mediated intracellular shift of potassium during the infusion
  - If cardiac arrest from hypokalemia is imminent, give an initial infusion of 2 mEq/min, followed by another 10 mEq IV over 5–10 min. Document in medical chart that rapid infusion is intentional owing to life-threatening situation. Once the patient is stabilized, reduce the infusion to gradual replacement[a]
- Asymptomatic
  - Increase dietary intake
    - Figs, dates, prunes, bananas, oranges, kiwis, and mangos

- Avocados, lima beans, and vegetables
- Beef, veal, and pork
○ Salt substitutes (usually with potassium phosphate)
○ Potassium chloride 20–40 mEq enterally daily
  - Adjust dose to maintain normokalemia
○ Consider concomitant utilization of a potassium-sparing diuretic (e.g., spironolactone, amiloride, and triamterene) if renal losses because of loop or thiazide diuretics

[a]Guidelines 2000 for Cardiopulmonary Resuscitation and Emergency Cardiovascular Care. *Circulation* 2000;102(8):I218.

Table 14.8
Management of Acute Hyperkalemia
(Serum Potassium ≥5.5 mEq/L)

Agent	*Comments*
Calcium gluconate (15–30 mL) of a 10% solution over 2–5 min (peripheral line) or Calcium chloride (5–10 mL) of a 10% solution over 2–5 min (central line)	• Administer if abnormal electrocardiogram (ECG) or if serum potassium is >7 mEq/L • Repeat every 30 min until ECG normalizes • Avoid if suspected digitalis toxicity. If severe symptomatic hyperkalemia and concomitant digoxin toxicity, treat with Digibind prior to infusing calcium if time permits • Onset: 1–2 min • Duration: 10–30 min
Sodium bicarbonate 45 mEq IV over 5 min	• Administer if abnormal ECG or pre-existing nonorganic metabolic acidosis • Onset: 30–60 min • Duration: 2–6 h

(Continued)

Table 14.8 *(Continued)*

Agent	Comments
	• Can repeat dose in 30 min if necessary
Regular insulin 10 units IV over 5–10 min	• Onset: 15–30 min • Duration: 2–6 h
Dextrose 50% 50–100 mL IV over 5–10 min	• Withhold if blood glucose >250 mg/dL • Onset: 15–30 min • Duration: 2–6 h
Furosemide 20–80 mg (1 mg/kg) IV over 2–5 min	• Onset: 15 min • Duration: 6 h
Albuterol 10–20 mg nebulized over 10 min	• Second-line pharmacotherapy • Onset: 30 min • Duration: 1–6 h
Sodium polystyrene sulfonate 15–60 g in 20% sorbitol suspension enterally. As an enema, prepare 50 g in 70% sorbitol plus 100 mL tap water. This solution should be retained for 30–60 min	• Enteral route more effective • Onset: 1–2 h • Duration: variable • Repeat every 4–6 h as needed
Hemodialysis cession (3–4 h)	• Use in patients with end-stage renal disease or if life-threatening emergency • Onset: immediate • Duration: variable

Notes:
1. Treatment depends on degree of hyperkalemia and presence/severity of signs and symptoms (sometimes irrespective of actual serum potassium level). *Mild:* 5.5–6 mEq/L—furosemide and sodium polystyrene sulfonate. *Moderate:* 6.1–7 mEq/L—insulin, glucose, sodium bicarbonate,

albuterol, furosemide, and sodium polystyrene sulfonate. *Severe:* >7 mEq/L—calcium, insulin, glucose, sodium bicarbonate, albuterol, furosemide and sodium polystyrene sulfonate.

2. Monitor serum potassium levels every 2 h until normalizes.

Table 14.9
Management of Acute Hypomagnesemia
(Serum Magnesium <1.4 mEq/L)

- Evaluate etiology
  - Drug-induced may include:
    - Thiazides, loop diuretics
    - Aminoglycosides, amphotericin B
    - Cyclosporine, tacrolimus, foscarnet, pentamidine
    - Cisplatin, ethanol
- Symptomatic or severe (≤1 mEq/L)
  - Magnesium sulfate 1–2 g IV over 15–30 min, repeat as needed to correct serum magnesium level
  - If seizures are present, administer 2 g IV over 2–5 min
- Asymptomatic or level >1 mEq/L
  - Magnesium oxide 300 mg enterally tid-qid
  - Milk of magnesia 5 mL tid-qid
  - Adjust dose until serum magnesium normalizes
  - Cautious dosing in patients with renal dysfunction

TID-QID, three times daily-four times daily.

Table 14.10
Management of Acute Hypermagnesemia
(Serum Magnesium >2 mEq/L)

- Evaluate etiology
  - Drug-induced may include:
    - Magnesium administration (IV, enteral, and enemas)
      - Milk-alkali syndrome
    - Theophylline, lithium

- Symptomatic
  - ○ Calcium chloride (central line) 5–10 mL of a 10% solution or calcium gluconate (peripheral line) 15–30 mL of a 10% solution over 5–10 min
    - ■ Repeat every hour as needed
  - ○ Forced diuresis in patients with adequate renal function
    - ■ 0.9% saline
    - ■ Furosemide 1 mg/kg IV in one dose
      - □ Subsequent dosing based on clinical response
      - □ May cause hypocalcemia, which may worsen the signs and symptoms of hypomagnesemia
  - ○ Hemodialysis
  - ○ Supportive care
    - ■ Vasopressors, cardiac pacing and mechanical ventilation

---

Table 14.11
Management of Acute Hyponatremia
(Serum Sodium <135 mEq/L)

Determine serum osmolality
- Serum osmolality$_{mOsm/kg}$ = 2(Na$_{mEq/L}$) + glucose$_{mg/dL}$/18 + BUN$_{mg/dL}$/2.8 + Etoh$_{mg/dL}$/4.6

Isotonic hyponatremia (275–290 mOsm/kg)
- Pseudohyponatremia caused by hyperlipidemia or paraproteinemias
  - ○ If serum sodium is measured by flame photometry
  - ○ Uncommon today with the use of ion (sodium) specific electrodes

Hypertonic hyponatremia (>290 mOsm/kg)
- Excess effective osmoles in the extracellular fluid
  - ○ Hyperglycemic state or use of mannitol
    - ■ For every 100 mg/dL rise in serum glucose, the serum sodium decreases by 1.6 mEq/L

- ○ Suspect unmeasured osmoles if the osmolar gap is
  >15 mOsm/kg

Hypotonic hyponatremia (<275 mOsm/kg)
- Hypovolemic state
  - ○ Urine sodium <10 mEq/L considered extrarenal losses
    - Gastrointestinal–vomiting, nasogastric suctioning,
      and diarrhea
    - Skin: fever and burns
    - Third-spacing: sepsis and pancreatitis
  - ○ Urine sodium ≥20 mEq/L considered renal losses
    - Diuretic use
    - Adrenal insufficiency
    - Salt-wasting nephropathy
    - Cerebral salt-wasting syndrome
- Euvolemic state
  - ○ Urine osmolality <100 mOsm/kg (anti-diuretic hormone
    [ADH] suppressed)
    - Psychogenic polydipsia
    - Beer potomania syndrome or "tea and toast" diet
  - ○ Urine osmolality ≥100 mOsm/kg (ADH present)
    - SIADH (should distinguish between cerebral salt-wasting
      syndrome in which patients are volume-contracted)
      - □ Causes
        - ◆ Pulmonary disease, small-cell lung cancer, head trauma,
          stroke, central nervous system infections, pituitary surgery,
          prolactinoma, severe nausea, psychiatric disease, and
          postoperative state
        - ◆ Antipsychotics, bromocriptine, carbamazepine,
          chlorpropamide, cyclophosphamide, desmopressin,
          ecstasy, lamotrigine, monamine oxidase inhibitors,
          NSAIDs, oxcarbazepine, oxytocin, tricyclic antide-
          pressants, selective serotonin reuptake inhibitors,
          vasopressin, vinblastine, and vincristine
    - Hypothyroidism
    - Adrenal insufficiency
    - Reset osmostat

       □ Hypovolemia, pregnant state, tuberculosis
       □ Manage underlying condition
- Hypervolemic state
  - Urine sodium <10 mEq/L (sodium avid)
    - Chronic heart failure, cirrhosis, and nephrotic syndrome
  - Urine sodium ≥20 mEq/L
    - Renal failure

Management
- Depends on rapidity of onset and symptoms
  - Rapid onset symptomatic hyponatremia warrants aggressive therapy
  - Asymptomatic patients do not warrant aggressive therapy
    - Usual rate of correction ≤0.5 mEq/L/h
  - Avoid a serum sodium rise >8–12 mEq/L within 24 h to prevent precipitation of osmotic demyelination (i.e., central pontine and extrapontine myelinolysis)
    - Unless severe central nervous system symptoms of acute hyponatremia persist after this level of correction (rarely encountered)
  - Rule out adrenal insufficiency and hypothyroidism
- *Acute symptomatic* (usual serum sodium <120 mEq/L)
  - Address etiology and stop any offending medication
  - Regardless of volume status, treat with 0.9% or 3% saline (*see* below) until signs and symptoms resolve
  - The patient can be placed on fluid restriction once signs and symptoms have resolved
  - Raise the serum sodium at a rate of 1.5–2 mEq/L/h for the first 2–4 h in patients with severe symptoms (i.e., coma and seizures) or until symptoms resolve
  - Do not exceed a serum sodium rise >8–12 mEq/L within 24 h and >18 mEq/L within 48 h
    - A greater change in serum sodium may be required if severe signs/symptoms secondary to hyponatremia persist. Another exception may be hyponatremia occurring in the setting after transurethral resection of the prostate (TURP)

- ○ Monitor serum sodium every 2–4 h and urinary osmolality and sodium every 4–6 h for the first 24 h
- ○ Potassium is as osmotically active as sodium; therefore, the effect of potassium administration (in a hypokalemic patient) on sodium concentration and osmolality should be taken into consideration
- ○ Calculate sodium deficit (SD)
  - ■ SD = (120 mEq/L – patient's serum sodium) × (patient's weight in kg × Vd)
    - □ Vd for males = 0.6 L/kg
    - □ Vd for females = 0.5 L/kg
- ○ Example calculation
  - ■ A 65-yr-old male patient (70 kg) presents with serum sodium of 110 mEq/L and seizures. How much intravenous 3% saline should this patient receive?
    - □ Determine volume required
      - ◆ $(120 - 110) \times (0.6 \times 70 \text{ kg}) = 420$ mEq
      - ◆ 513 mEq/1000 mL = 420 mEq/x
        - ◇ $x = 819$ mL of 3% saline required to correct
    - □ Determine rate
      - ◆ 819 mL/10 mEq$_{(\Delta \text{ Na})}$ = x/1.5 mEq (maximum hourly increase)
        - ◇ $x = 123$ mL maximum per hour
        - ◇ Therefore initiate 3% saline at 120 mL/h
    - □ Seizures cease after a total of 2 h
      - ◆ At this point the patient received 240 mL of 3% saline
      - ◆ 819 mL – 240 mL = 579 mL remaining over 22 h
        - ◇ Therefore reduce rate to 25 mL/h for 22 h
- ○ Important to note that these formulas do not account for ongoing solute and water losses
- • Hypovolemic state
  - ○ Utilize 0.9% (isotonic) saline (154 mEq/L and 308 mOsm/L)
    - ■ May raise plasma sodium by 1–2 mEq/L of solution infused
- • Euvolemic state
  - ○ SIADH
    - ■ If urine osmolality is ≤300 mOsm/L, may use 0.9% saline if mild signs and symptoms (i.e., headache, nausea, vomiting, and weakness)

- If urine osmolality exceeds 300 mOsm/L, add a loop diuretic (e.g., furosemide 40 mg IV q6h) to 0.9% saline or use 3% saline (513 mEq/L and 1026 mOsm/L)
- Utilize 3% saline for severe signs and symptoms (i.e., altered mental status, coma, and seizures)
  □ 0.9% isotonic saline may *worsen* hyponatremia if urine osmolality is high
- Note, if asymptomatic, just restrict fluid to between 1000 and 1200 mL/d +/– high protein diet +/– sodium chloride (NaCl) tablets
○ Conivaptan may be utilized in carefully selected patients
  - Loading dose – 20 mg IV over 30 min × one dose. Evaluate response and need for additional doses or continuous IV infusion
  - The loading dose may be followed by a continuous IV infusion of 20 mg over 24 h. May titrate to a maximum of 40 mg/d if inadequate response. Total duration of therapy not to exceed 4 d
- Hypervolemic state
  ○ Fluid restriction to between 1000 and 1200 mL/d
  ○ Utilize a loop diuretic
  ○ Utilize 3% saline (513 mEq/L and 1026 mOsm/L) plus loop diuretic for severe signs and symptoms

---

Table 14.12
Management of Acute Hypernatremia
(Serum Sodium >145 mEq/L)

Hypovolemic hypernatremia (loss of water and sodium [water > sodium])
- Renal losses
  ○ Diuretics, mannitol, and glucosuria
- Extrarenal losses
  ○ Excessive sweating, osmotic diarrhea, vomiting, nasogastric suctioning, and respiratory
- Management
  ○ If postural hypotension present

- Normal saline
  - □ Change to hypotonic saline or dextrose 5% in water to correct free water deficit once intravascular replete
- Primarily water depletion
  - Hypotonic saline or dextrose 5% in water

Euvolemic hypernatremia (loss of water)
- Renal losses
  - Central or nephrogenic diabetes insipidus
- Extrarenal losses
  - Insensible pulmonary and skin losses
- Management
  - Water replacement as dextrose 5% in water
  - Central diabetes insipidus
    - Vasopressin
      - □ 5–10 units SQ q6-12 h (dosage range 5–60 units/d)
      - □ Continuous IV infusion regimen: 0.0005 units/kg/h; double dose as needed every 30 min to a maximum of 0.01 units/kg/h
    - Desmopressin
      - □ 2–4 mcg IV/SQ daily administered as a single daily dose or in two divided doses
      - □ 10–40 mcg in 1–3 divided doses intranasally daily
    - Notes
      - □ Adjust morning and evening doses separately to consider diurnal variation in water excretion
      - □ Adjust dose based on urine output, urine osmolality, and serum sodium
  - Nephrogenic diabetes insipidus
    - Sodium restriction (<2000 mg/d)
      - □ Consider dietary, fluid, and medication sodium sources
    - Hydrochlorothiazide 25 mg enterally q12-24 h (may work in central diabetes insipidus)
    - Amiloride 5–10 mg enterally daily if lithium-related
    - Indomethacin 50 mg enterally q8h (may work in central diabetes insipidus)

Hypervolemic hypernatremia (water and sodium gain
[sodium > water])
- Sodium overload
  - ○ Example, sodium-rich medications, sodium bicarbonate, hypertonic IV fluids, nutrition, enemas, dialysis, plasma products (sodium citrate content)
- Mineralocorticoid excess
- Management
  - ○ Loop diuretics (e.g., furosemide 40 mg IV q6h) and water replacement as dextrose 5% in water

Calculating water deficit and general management
principles
- Water deficit = Vd (weight in kg) × ([patient's serum sodium/140] – 1)
  - ○ Vd for males = 0.6 L/kg
  - ○ Vd for females = 0.5 L/kg
- Administer half of deficit over 24 h, then remainder over next 1–2 d
- Goal should be a serum sodium <145 mEq/L
  - ○ Monitor serum sodium every 2–3 h over the first 24 h
- Serum sodium in acute-onset hypernatremia may be lowered by 1 mEq/L/h
- Serum sodium in slow-onset hypernatremia may be lowered by 0.5 mEq/L/h
- Sodium decrease should not be >12 mEq/L in the first 24 h
- Rapid correction may result in cerebral edema, seizures, central pontine myelinolysis, or death
- In the setting of hyperglycemia, use the corrected serum sodium to estimate free water deficit
  - ○ Add 1.6 mEq/L to the measured serum sodium for every 100 mg/dL rise in serum glucose above 200 mg/dL
- The above water deficit equation does not take into consideration continuous free water losses (i.e., insensible, renal, or gastrointestinal)

Table 14.13
Management of Acute Hypophosphatemia (<2 mg/dL)

- Intravenous pharmacotherapy
  - Intravenous formulations contain either sodium 4 mEq/mL or potassium 4.4 mEq/mL with 3 mmol/mL phosphate
  - Symptomatic and severe hypophosphatemia (≤1 mg/dL)
    - 0.25 mmol/kg (ideal body weight) over 6 h, repeat as necessary
  - Symptomatic and moderate hypophosphatemia (between 1 and 2 mg/dL)
    - 0.15 mmol/kg (ideal body weight) over 6 h, repeat as necessary
  - Monitor for hypernatremia or hyperkalemia, hypocalcemia, and metastatic soft tissue deposition of calcium-phosphate crystals
- Enteral supplementation
  - Neutra-Phos (Na-7 mEq, K-7 mEq, and PO_4^- 250 mg) per packet
  - Neutra-Phos K (K-14.25 mEq and PO_4^- 250 mg) per capsule
  - K-Phos Neutral (Na-13 mEq, K-1.27 mEq, and PO_4^- 250 mg) per tablet
  - Initiate pharmacotherapy with 1–2 g/d in three divided doses
    - Reduce dose and monitor carefully in patients with renal impairment

Table 14.14
Management of Hyperphosphatemia (>5 mg/dL)

- Severe hyperphosphatemia, presenting as hypocalcemia and tetany should be treated with hemodialysis and possibly careful intravenous calcium administration (*see* management of hypocalcemia)
- Dietary and phosphorus-containing medication restriction
  - Protein restrict to 0.6–0.8 g/kg/d
  - Foods high in phosphorus include:

- ■ Diary products, cola beverages, beer, dried beans, peanut butter
  - ○ Avoid phosphate-containing laxatives (e.g., Fleet's Phospho-Soda), sodium or potassium phosphate solutions, avoid hypervitaminosis D
- Phosphate binders
  - ○ Administer just before or with a meal to maximize effects
  - ○ Calcium salts (acetate, carbonate, and citrate)
    - ■ Dose of elemental calcium should not exceed 1.5–2 g/d and plasma calcium levels should not exceed 9.5 mg/dL (to avoid coronary artery calcification resulting from excess calcium)
    - ■ First-line agents (except when patient has concomitant hypercalcemia)
    - ■ Titrate dose to achieve normophosphatemia
    - ■ Calcium carbonate requires an acidic medium for solubility
      - □ H_2-receptor antagonists and proton pump inhibitors may affect solubility
    - ■ Calcium citrate should not be administered with aluminum-containing compounds. Concomitant administration may increase systemic bioavailability of aluminum and predispose to toxicity
    - ■ May place patients at risk for vascular calcification
      - □ Combine with sevelamer if high-dose calcium salts are required to correct hyperphosphatemia
- Sevelamer
  - ○ Initiate therapy with 800 mg enterally tid with meals (up to 1600 mg tid)
  - ○ Use in patients who have concomitant hypercalcemia and/or a calcium/phosphate product >55
- Aluminum-containing solutions
  - ○ Avoid concomitant use with citrate-containing products
  - ○ Avoid chronic use (>1 mo)
    - ■ If chronic use is required in patients with end-stage renal disease, monitor serum aluminum concentrations every 3 mo

Table 14.15
Management of Acute Primary Metabolic Acidosis
(pH < 7.35)

Determine etiology (bicarbonate loss or nonvolatile acid gain)
- Anion gap metabolic acidosis (AG = Na − [Cl + HCO$_3$])
  - MUDPILES
    - Methanol
    - Uremia
    - Diabetic ketoacidosis
      - Alcoholic or starvation ketoacidosis
    - Paraldehyde
    - Isoniazid or iron (lactic acidosis)
    - Lactic acidosis
      - Type A (associated with tissue hypoxia)
        - Cardiogenic/distributive/obstructive/hypovolemic shock, carbon monoxide poisoning, severe hypoxemia, severe anemia, and seizures
        - Limb and intestinal ischemia
      - Type B (deranged oxidative metabolism)
        - Acute leukemia, acute lymphoma, short-bowel syndrome, liver disease (decreased clearance), diabetes mellitus, mitochondrial disease, and congenital enzyme deficiencies
        - Metformin, salicylates, iron, isoniazid, and antiretrovirals
        - Cyanide poisoning (e.g., nitroprusside), methanol, ethanol, and ethylene glycol
    - Ethylene glycol
    - Salicylate
    - Other
      - Theophylline and toluene
- Hyperchloremic (nonanion gap) metabolic acidosis
  - Consumption/loss of bicarbonate
    - Gastrointestinal losses (e.g., diarrhea, fistula, ileostomy, ureterosigmoidostomy)
    - Dilutional (administration of nonalkali fluids [i.e., normal saline, D5W])

- Renal losses (e.g., proximal [Type II] renal tubular acidosis [RTA])
  - Complication of carbonic anhydrase inhibitor or topiramate pharmacotherapy
  - Heavy metals (e.g., cadmium, mercury, and lead)
  - Outdated tetracycline (Fanconi's syndrome)
  - Nephrotic syndrome, multiple myeloma, Wilson's disease, and amyloidosis
  - Responsive to sodium bicarbonate 10–15 mEq/kg/d
  - Decreased renal acid excretion
    - Distal (Type I) RTA—hypokalemic (secondary hypoaldosteronism)
      - Systemic lupus erythematosus, Sjogren's syndrome, multiple myeloma, obstructive uropathy, cirrhosis, and sickle cell disease
      - Hypercalcemia, amphotericin B, and toluene
      - Responsive to sodium bicarbonate 1–3 mEq/kg/d
    - Distal (Type IV) RTA—hyperkalemic (hyporeninemic hypoaldosteronism)
      - Diabetic or HIV nephropathy, analgesic abuse nephropathy, cyclosporine nephropathy, and chronic interstitial nephritis
      - Pharmacologically exacerbated by angiotensin converting enzyme inhibitors, angiotensin receptor blockers, β-adrenergic blockers, dihydropyridine calcium channel blockers, spironolactone, eplerenone, heparin, and NSAIDs
      - Manage hyperkalemia (dietary restriction) or responsive to sodium bicarbonate 1–3 mEq/kg/d
        - May need fludrocortisone, kayexelate, or loop diuretic pharmacotherapy
  - Accumulation of exogenous acid
    - Ammonium chloride, hydrochloric acid, arginine monohydrochloride, and toluene
    - Parenteral nutrition (amino acid salts) and arginine

Management
- Address etiology
- Sodium bicarbonate
  - May be utilized in:
    - Severe metabolic acidosis (pH < 7.2 or serum HCO_3 < 8 mEq/L)
    - Bicarbonate losing states
    - Salicylate toxicity
    - Convincing data in lactic acidosis is lacking
      - Manage underlying etiology
      - Utilize if associated symptomatic hyperkalemia
      - May be warranted in very severe metabolic acidosis
  - Goal:
    - pH > 7.2 or HCO_3 between 8 and 10 mEq/L
    - Do not normalize these parameters
    - These goals may minimize an "overshoot" metabolic alkalosis
      - Remember that ketoacids and lactic acid are metabolized to bicarbonate
  - Calculate bicarbonate deficit (BD) to determine dose
    - BD = (8 – patient's serum HCO_3) × 0.5 (ideal body weight)
    - Administer as an intravenous infusion over 1–4 h
    - Follow-up with arterial blood gases to determine correction and need for additional sodium bicarbonate therapy
- Tromethamine (THAM)
  - Acts as a proton acceptor
    - Combines with H^+ from carbonic acid to form bicarbonate and a cationic buffer
    - Nonbicarbonate buffer
      - Does not increase carbon dioxide production
    - May increase intracellular pH
    - Contraindicated in renal failure
    - Dose of 0.3 *N* THAM (mL) = 1.1 ([ABW in kg] × [goal HCO_3 – patient's HCO_3]) administered intravenously >1–6 h using a large peripheral vein or central vein
      - Additional doses determined by base deficit

- Contraindicated in patients who are anuric or uremic or have chronic respiratory acidosis or salicylate toxicity
- Monitor for hyperkalemia and hypoglycemia

Table 14.16
Management of Acute Primary Metabolic Alkalosis (pH > 7.45)

Determine etiology (loss of H^+ [or chloride-rich fluid] or gain of HCO_3^- rich fluid)

- Chloride-responsive or volume-depleted states (urinary chloride concentration <10 mEq/L)
  - Diuretic pharmacotherapy (renal H^+/chloride losses/2° hyperaldosteronism, renal ammoniagenesis)
    - Example, loop diuretics and thiazides
  - Gastrointestinal losses (H^+/chloride losses)
    - Vomiting, nasogastric suctioning, and chloride (secretory) diarrhea (villous adenoma or laxative abuse)
  - Perspiratory losses in patients with cystic fibrosis
  - Mild-to-moderate potassium depletion (renal ammoniagenesis)
  - Posthypercapnea
- Chloride-unresponsive (urinary chloride concentration >20 mEq/L)
  - Excess mineralocorticoid activity (renal H^+ losses, hypokalemia-induced renal ammoniagenesis)
    - Example, Bartter's or Gitelman's syndrome, Cushing's syndrome, hyperaldosteronism (1° or 2°), and Liddle's syndrome
    - Black licorice (glycyrrhizic acid) consumption
  - Severe potassium (K < 2 mEq/L) and magnesium (Mg < 1 mEq/L) depletion (renal ammoniagenesis, renal H^+ losses, and stimulate renal bicarbonate reabsorption)
- Indeterminent
  - Excessive alkali administration
    - Bicarbonate, acetate, citrate, and lactate
    - Milk-alkali syndrome
  - High-dose penicillin therapy (e.g., ticarcillin)

Management

- Address etiology
- Chloride-responsive or volume-depleted states
  - Intravenous normal saline (to address volume depletion)
  - Potassium, magnesium, and calcium chloride replacement if warranted
  - Upper gastrointestinal losses
    - H_2-receptor antagonists, proton pump inhibitors
  - If patient is adequately hydrated, potassium-repleted, or volume intolerant
    - Acetazolamide 250–500 mg IV/enterally bid
      - Rarely, may lead to a small rise in PCO_2 in patients with chronic respiratory acidosis
  - If alkalosis persists or if pH > 7.6 or HCO_3 >45 mEq/L
    - Hydrochloric acid
      - HCl dose in mEq = 0.5 (IBW) × (patient's serum HCO_3 – 40)
      - 0.1 N HCl = 100 mEq/L
      - 0.2 N HCl = 200 mEq/L
      - Administer through a central line at ≤0.2 mEq/kg/h
        - Decrease infusion rate in the presence of respiratory compensation to avoid respiratory acidosis
      - Discontinue infusion when the arterial pH reaches 7.5
    - Arginine monohydrochloride
      - 10 g/h continuous IV infusion
      - Discontinue infusion when the arterial pH reaches 7.5
      - Do not administer in patients in septic shock
    - Ammonia chloride has a limited role
  - Hemodialysis using a low-bicarbonate dialysate
- Chloride-unresponsive
  - Potassium chloride replacement
  - Excessive mineralocorticoid activity
    - Decrease dose or change corticosteroid to one with less mineralocorticoid activity (e.g., dexamethasone)
    - Bartter's or Gitelman's syndrome
      - Spironolactone, amiloride, and triamterene
    - Liddle's syndrome
      - Amiloride, triamterene
    - Decrease/eliminate exogenous alkali administration

Table 14.17
Dosing of Selected Intravenous Anti-Infectives in Patients Receiving Continuous Renal Replacement Therapy

Antimicrobial	CVVH	CVVHD/CVVHDF
• Acyclovir	• 5–7.5 mg/kg q24h	• 5–7.5 mg/kg q24h
• Ampicillin/ sulbactam	• 1.5–3 g q12h	• 1.5–3 g q8h
• Aztreonam	• 1–2 g q12h	• 2 g q12h
• Cefazolin	• 1–2 g q12h	• 2 g q12h
• Cefepime	• 1–2 g q12h	• 2 g q12h
• Cefotaxime	• 1–2 g q12h	• 2 g q12h
• Ceftazidime	• 1–2 g q12h	• 2 g q12h
• Ciprofloxacin	• 200 mg q12h	• 400 mg q12h
• Colistin	• 2.5 mg/kg q48h	• 2.5 mg/kg q48h
• Daptomycin	• 4 or 6 mg/kg q48h	• 4 or 6 mg/kg q48h
• Fluconazole	• 200–400 mg q24h	• 400–800 mg q24h
• Imipenem/ cilastatin[a]	• 500 mg q8h	• 500 mg q6-8 h
• Levofloxacin	• 250–500 mg q24h	• 250–500 mg q24h
• Meropenem	• 500–1000 mg q12h	• 500–1000 mg q8-12h
• Oxacillin	• 2 g q4-6 h	• 2 g q4-6h
• Penicillin	• 4 million units q8h	• 4 million units q6h
• Piperacillin/ tazobactam	• 2.25g q6h	• 2.25–3.375 g q6h
• Vancomycin	• 10–15 mg/kg q24h	• 15 mg/kg q24h

CVVH, continuous venovenous hemofiltration; CVVHD, continuous venovenous hemodialysis; CVVHDF, continuous venovenous hemodiafiltration.

Recommendations based on ultrafiltration and dialysate flow rates of 1 L/h.

CID 2005;41:1159–1166.

[a]Adjust dose of imipenem/cilastatin based on body weight (refer to package insert).

Index

A

ABW. *See* Actual body weight (ABW)
ACE-I. *See* Angiotensin converting enzyme inhibitors (ACE-I)
Acetazolamide
    acute primary metabolic acidosis, 181
Acetylcysteine
    contrast-induced nephropathy prevention, 156
    ICU toxicological emergencies, 94
ACLS. *See* Advance cardiac life support (ACLS)
Acquired Torsades de Pointes, 43–44
Actual body weight (ABW), 137
Acute aortic dissection, 46
Acute asthma exacerbations, 151–154
Acute cerebrovascular accident
    blood pressure management, 56–57
    supportive care, 55
Acute coronary syndrome, 46
Acute decompensated heart failure, 35–36
Acute hypercalcemia, 162–164
Acute hyperkalemia, 165–166
Acute hypermagnesemia, 167–168
Acute hypernatremia, 172–174
Acute hypocalcemia, 161–162
Acute hypokalemia, 164–165
Acute hypomagnesemia, 167
Acute hyponatremia, 168–172
Acute hypophosphatemia, 175
Acute nonvariceal upper gastrointestinal bleeding, 109–110
Acute primary metabolic acidosis, 177–181
Acute renal failure, 47, 157
Acute uremic bleeding, 159
Acyclovir
    intravenous dosage, 182

Adenosine
    dosage, 11
Advance cardiac life support (ACLS), 1
    code algorithms, 1–20
    common drugs utilized, 11–18
    pulseless arrest algorithm, 1
Agranulocytosis, 119
Albumin
    hepatorenal syndrome, 115
Albuterol
    acute asthma exacerbations, 151
    acute hyperkalemia, 166
    nebulization in anaphylaxis/anaphylactoid reactions, 20
Alcohol withdrawal, 143–145
Aldosterone receptor blockade
    ST-elevation myocardial infarction, 32
Alteplase (tPA)
    inclusion and exclusion criteria for cerebrovascular accident
        indication, 57–58
    induced intracranial hemorrhage, 61
    protocol for cerebrovascular accident indication, 60,61
    pulmonary embolism, 51
    ST-elevation myocardial infarction, 28
Amikacin
    therapeutic drug monitoring in ICU, 90–91
Amiloride
    nephrogenic diabetes insipidus, 173
Amiodarone, 39
    dosage, 11–12
    narrow complex stable supraventricular tachycardia, 7, 8
    stable atrial fibrillation/atrial flutter, 6
    stable ventricular tachycardia, 8, 9, 12
Ampicillin
    intravenous dosage, 182
Analgesia
    critical care, 71–72, 73
Anaphylaxis/anaphylactoid reactions
    pharmacological management, 19–20
Anemia
    aplastic, 119
    hemolytic, 120
    megaloblastic, 120

Angina
    unstable
        and non-ST elevation myocardial infarction, 23–24
        short-term risk of death or nonfatal myocardial infarction
            with, 22–23
Angioedema, 101
Angiotensin converting enzyme inhibitors (ACE-I)
    ST-elevation myocardial infarction, 32
    unstable angina and non-ST elevation myocardial infarction,
        26–27
Angiotensin receptor blockers (ARB)
    ST-elevation myocardial infarction, 32
Anion gap metabolic acidosis, 177
Antiarrhythmics
    Vaughan Williams classification, 38–39
Antihistamines
    anaphylaxis/anaphylactoid reactions, 19
Antithrombotic pharmacotherapy, 40–41
Aortic dissection
    acute, 46
Aplastic anemia, 119
ARB. *See* Angiotensin receptor blockers (ARB)
Argatroban
    heparin-induced thrombocytopenia, 121
Arginine monohydrochloride
    acute primary metabolic acidosis, 181
Ascites, 112
    refractory, 113
    tense, 112–113
Aspirin
    ST-elevation myocardial infarction, 29
    unstable angina and non-ST elevation myocardial
        infarction, 23
Asthma
    acute exacerbations, 151–154
Asystole algorithm, 3
Atenolol
    ST-elevation myocardial infarction, 30–31
    unstable angina and non-ST elevation myocardial
    infarction, 25
Atracurium
    ICU, 79–80

Atrial fibrillation
        antithrombotic pharmacotherapy, 40–41
        stable
            management, 5–7
Atrial flutter. *See* Atrial fibrillation
Atropine
        asystole algorithm, 3
        bradycardia algorithm, 4
        dosage, 12, 18
        pulseless electrical activity algorithm, 3
Autoimmune drug-induced hepatotoxicity, 117
Aztreonam
        intravenous dosage, 182

B

Barbiturate
        synchronized cardioversion algorithm for symptomatic
        tachycardia management, 10
Benzodiazepine
        alcohol withdrawal, 143
Beta-adrenergic blockers, 38
        stable atrial fibrillation/atrial flutter, 5
        stable ventricular tachycardia, 9
        ST-elevation myocardial infarction, 30–31
        unstable angina and non-ST elevation myocardial
        infarction, 25
Bisphosphonates
        acute hypercalcemia, 163
Body weight
        actual, 137
        ideal, 137
Bradycardia
        algorithm, 3–4
        atropine, 4, 12
        epinephrine, 15

C

Calcitonin salmon
        acute hypercalcemia, 163
Calcium carbonate
        acute hypocalcemia, 162
        hyperphosphatemia, 176

Calcium channel blockers
    ST-elevation myocardial infarction, 32
Calcium chloride
    acute hyperkalemia, 165
    acute hypermagnesemia, 168
    acute hypocalcemia, 161
Calcium citrate
    hyperphosphatemia, 176
Calcium gluconate
    acute hyperkalemia, 165
    acute hypocalcemia, 161–162, 162
Calcium lactate
    acute hypocalcemia, 162
Calories
    daily needs, 138
Captopril
    hypertensive urgencies, 47
Carbamazepine
    therapeutic drug monitoring in ICU, 91
Carbohydrates, 139
Cardiac arrest
    amiodarone, 11
    atropine, 12
    epinephrine, 14
    lidocaine, 16
    magnesium sulfate, 16
    sodium bicarbonate, 16–17
Cardiovascular, 21–54
Catecholamine
    crisis, 46
    extravasation, 47
Cefazolin
    intravenous dosage, 182
Cefepime
    intravenous dosage, 182
Ceftazidime
    intravenous dosage, 182
Cerebrovascular, 55–64
    accident
        alteplase, 57–58, 60–61
        blood pressure management, 56–57
        supportive care, 55

Chelating agents
   acute hypercalcemia, 163
Chlordiazepoxide
   alcohol withdrawal, 144
Chlorothiazide
   acute renal failure, 158
Cholestasis
   drug-induced hepatotoxicity, 117
Chordiazepoxide
   propylene glycol content, 86
Chronic obstructive pulmonary disease (COPD), 149–150
Cilastatin
   intravenous dosage, 182
Cimetidine
   methemoglobinemia, 124
   stress-related mucosal damage prophylaxis, 88
Ciprofloxacin
   intravenous dosage, 182
   VAP, 128
Cirrhosis, 111–112
Cisatracurium
   ICU, 79
CIWA-Ar. *See* Clinical institute withdrawal assessment for alcohol
   scale (CIWA-Ar)
Clinical institute withdrawal assessment for alcohol scale (CIWA-Ar),
   143
Clinical pulmonary infection score (CPIS), 128–129
Clonidine
   hypertensive urgencies, 47
Clopidogrel
   ST-elevation myocardial infarction, 29
   unstable angina and non-ST elevation myocardial infarction,
      23–24
Code algorithms
   ACLS, 1–20
Colistin
   intravenous dosage, 182
Conivaptan
   hyponatremia, 172
   propylene glycol content, 86
Conjugated estrogen
   acute uremic bleeding, 159

Continuous renal replacement therapy
  intravenous anti-infectives, 182
Contrast-induced nephropathy prevention, 155–156
Convulsive status epilepticus, 131–132
COPD. *See* Chronic obstructive pulmonary disease (COPD)
Corticosteroids
  septic shock, 69–70
Cough
  drug-induced, 154
CPIS. *See* Clinical pulmonary infection score (CPIS)
Critical care, 65–99
  analgesia, 71–72, 73
  delirium, 71–72, 74
  diarrhea, 110–111
  drug utilization principles, 65–66
  erythropoietin and PRBC, 83–85
  fever
    causes, 125
    drug-induced, 87–88
  sedation, 71–72
  therapeutic drug monitoring, 90–91
  toxicological emergency antidotes, 94–99
Cryoprecipitate
  acute uremic bleeding, 159
Crystalloid/colloid
  acute decompensated heart failure, 35
Cyanokit
  ICU toxicological emergencies, 99
Cyproheptadine
  serotonin syndrome, 146

D

Daily caloric needs, 138
Daily protein needs, 138
Dalteparin
  deep vein thrombosis, 50
  pulmonary embolism, 52
  unstable angina and non-ST elevation myocardial
    infarction, 25
Dantrolene
  neuroleptic malignant syndrome, 148

Daptomycin
     intravenous dosage, 182
Death
     short-term risk of, 22–23
Decompensated heart failure, 35–36
Deep vein thrombosis, 49–50
Delirium
     critical care, 71–72, 74
          confusion assessment diagnosis, 76–78
Dermatological reactions
     drug-induced, 101–102
Dermatology, 101–102
Desmopressin
     acute uremic bleeding, 159
     euvolemic hypernatremia, 173
Dexmedetomidine
     critical care, 72
Dextrose
     acute hyperkalemia, 166
     convulsive status epilepticus, 132
Diabetes insipidus, 173
Diabetic ketoacidosis, 103–105
Diarrhea
     causes in ICU, 110–111
Diazepam
     alcohol withdrawal, 144
     convulsive status epilepticus, 132
     propylene glycol content, 86
     synchronized cardioversion algorithm for symptomatic
         tachycardia management, 10
Digibind
     ICU toxicological emergencies, 95
Digoxin
     dosage, 13–14
     narrow complex stable supraventricular tachycardia, 7
     propylene glycol content, 86
     stable atrial fibrillation/atrial flutter, 6
     therapeutic drug monitoring in ICU, 91
Diltiazem, 39
     dosage, 14
     narrow complex stable supraventricular
         tachycardia, 7, 8

stable atrial fibrillation/atrial flutter, 5, 6
ST-elevation myocardial infarction, 32
Diphenhydramine
anaphylaxis/anaphylactoid reactions, 19
Disopyramide, 38
Dobutamine
acute decompensated heart failure, 36, 37
septic shock, 68–69
Docusate sodium
ST-elevation myocardial infarction, 33
Dofelitide, 39
Dopamine
acute decompensated heart failure, 36
bradycardia algorithm, 4
septic shock, 68
Drotrecogin-alpha
septic shock, 69–70
Drug-induced dermatological reactions, 101–102
Drug-induced fever, 87–88
Drug-induced hematological disorders, 119–120
Drug-induced hepatotoxicity, 117–118
Drug-induced pancreatitis, 118
Drug-induced pulmonary disease, 154–155
Drug-induced renal disease, 159–160
Drug-nutrient interactions, 141

E

Elevated international normalized ratio with warfarin, 52–54
Encephalopathy, 113–114
Endocrinology, 103–108
Enoxaparin
deep vein thrombosis, 50
unstable angina and non-ST elevation myocardial
infarction, 25
Enteral nutrition
minimizing aspiration during, 142
Eosinophilic pulmonary infiltration
drug-induced, 154
Epinephrine, 15
acquired Torsades de Pointes, 44
anaphylaxis/anaphylactoid reactions, 20

asystole algorithm, 3
bradycardia algorithm, 4
dosage, 14–15, 18
pulseless electrical activity algorithm, 3
septic shock, 68
ventricular fibrillation/pulseless ventricular tachycardia
    algorithm, 2
Erythema multiforme, 101
Erythromycin
minimizing aspiration during enteral nutrition, 142
Erythropoietin
critically ill patients, 83–85
Esmolol
dosage, 15
narrow complex stable supraventricular tachycardia, 7, 8
propylene glycol content, 86
stable atrial fibrillation/atrial flutter, 6
thyrotoxic crisis, 107
Esomeprazole
stress-related mucosal damage prophylaxis, 88
Estrogen
acute uremic bleeding, 159
Etidronate
acute hypercalcemia, 163
Etomidate
propylene glycol content, 86
synchronized cardioversion algorithm for symptomatic
    tachycardia management, 10
Euvolemic hypernatremia, 173

F

Famotidine
anaphylaxis/anaphylactoid reactions, 19
stress-related mucosal damage prophylaxis, 88
Fentanyl
critical care, 73
Fever
causes, 125
drug-induced, 87–88
Fibrate
ST-elevation myocardial infarction, 33
unstable angina and non-ST elevation myocardial infarction, 27

Fibrinolytic therapy with ST-elevation myocardial infarction
    contraindications, 34–35
Fibrosis
    drug-induced hepatotoxicity, 117
Flecainide, 38
    stable atrial fibrillation/atrial flutter, 6
Fluconazole
    intravenous dosage, 182
Flumazenil
    ICU toxicological emergencies, 95–96
Fosphenytoin
    convulsive status epilepticus, 133
    therapeutic drug monitoring in ICU, 92–93
Furosemide
    acute decompensated heart failure, 35, 36
    acute hypercalcemia, 163
    acute hyperkalemia, 166
    acute hypermagnesemia, 168
    acute renal failure, 157
    ascites, 112

G

Gallium nitrate
    acute hypercalcemia, 163
Gastrointestinal bleeding
    acute nonvariceal upper, 109–110
Gastrointestinal disorders, 109–118
Gentamicin
    therapeutic drug monitoring in ICU, 91–92
Glomerular disease
    drug-induced, 159
Glucagon
    ICU toxicological emergencies, 96
Glucocorticoids
    acute hypercalcemia, 163
Glycoprotein IIb/IIIa inhibitors
    unstable angina and non-ST elevation myocardial infarction, 24

H

Haloperidol
    delirium
        critical care, 74

Heart failure
    acute decompensated, 35–36
Heart valves
    antithrombotic pharmacotherapy, 42
Hematological disorders
    drug-induced, 119–120
Hematology, 119–124
Hemolysis, 119
Hemolytic anemia, 120
Heparin. *See also* Low molecular weight heparin (LMWH)
    deep vein thrombosis, 49–50
    pulmonary embolism, 51
    unfractionated
        ST-elevation myocardial infarction, 29
        unstable angina and non-ST elevation myocardial
            infarction, 24–25
    venous thromboembolism prevention in ICU, 48–49
Heparin-induced thrombocytopenia, 121–122
Hepatic encephalopathy, 113–114
Hepatorenal syndrome, 114–116
    albumin, 115
Hepatotoxicity
    drug-induced, 117–118
        autoimmune, 117
Histamine$_2$-receptor antagonists
    acute nonvariceal upper gastrointestinal bleeding, 110
    anaphylaxis/anaphylactoid reactions, 19–20
Hospital-acquired pneumonia
    management, 126–127
    prevention, 125–126
Hydralazine
    propylene glycol content, 86
Hydrochloric acid
    acute primary metabolic acidosis, 181
Hydrochlorothiazide
    nephrogenic diabetes insipidus, 173
Hydrocortisone
    anaphylaxis/anaphylactoid reactions, 20
    myxedema coma, 108
    septic shock, 69–70
    thyrotoxic crisis, 107
Hydromorphone
    critical care, 73

Hydroxocobalamine
    ICU toxicological emergencies, 99
Hypercalcemia
    acute, 162–164
Hyperchloremic (non-anion gap) metabolic acidosis, 177–178
Hyperglycemic hyperosmolar nonketotic syndrome, 105–106
Hyperkalemia
    acute, 165–166
Hypermagnesemia
    acute, 167–168
Hypernatremia
    acute, 172–174
    euvolemic, 173
    hypervolemic, 174
    hypovolemic, 172–173
Hyperphosphatemia, 175–176
Hypertension, 62–63
Hypertensive crises, 44–47
Hypertensive emergency, 44–46
Hypertensive encephalopathy, 46–47
Hypertensive urgency, 45
Hyperthermia, 82–83
Hypertonic hyponatremia, 168–169
Hypervolemic hypernatremia, 174
Hypocalcemia, 161–162
Hypokalemia, 164–165
Hypomagnesemia, 167
Hyponatremia
    acute, 168–172
    hypertonic, 168–169
    hypotonic, 169
Hypophosphatemia, 175
Hypotonic hyponatremia, 169
Hypovolemic hypernatremia, 172–173

I

Ibutelide, 39
IBW. *See* Ideal body weight (IBW)
ICU. *See* Intensive care unit (ICU)
Ideal body weight (IBW), 137
Imipenem
    intravenous dosage, 182

Indomethacin
    nephrogenic diabetes insipidus, 173
Induced intracranial hemorrhage
    alteplase (tPA), 61
Infectious disease, 125–129
INR. *See* International normalized ratio (INR)
Insulin
    acute hyperkalemia, 166
    diabetic ketoacidosis, 104
    hyperglycemic hyperosmolar nonketotic syndrome,106
    ST-elevation myocardial infarction, 33
Intensive care unit (ICU). *See also* Critical care
    atracurium, 79–80
    and diarrhea, 110–111
    neuromuscular blockers, 79–80
    pancuronium, 79
    therapeutic drug monitoring, 90–94
    toxicological emergency antidotes, 94–99
    venous thromboembolism prevention, 48–49
International normalized ratio (INR)
    elevated with warfarin, 52–54
Interstitial nephritis, 159
Intracranial hemorrhage, 61
Intracranial hypertension management, 62–63
Isoproterenol
    acquired Torsades de Pointes, 44
    dosage, 15

K

Ketoacidosis, 103–105

L

Labetolol
    acute cerebrovascular accident blood pressure
        management, 57
    hypertensive urgencies, 47
Lactulose
    hepatic encephalopathy, 113
Lansoprazole
    stress-related mucosal damage prophylaxis, 88
Left ventricular failure, 46

Lepirudin
    heparin-induced thrombocytopenia, 121
Levofloxacin
    intravenous dosage, 182
Levothyroxine
    myxedema coma, 108
Lidocaine, 38
    acquired Torsades de Pointes, 44
    dosage, 16, 18
    stable ventricular tachycardia, 8, 9
    therapeutic drug monitoring in ICU, 92
Linezolid
    VAP, 127
Liothyronine
    myxedema coma, 108
Lipids, 139
LMWH. *See* Low molecular weight heparin (LMWH)
Loop diuretics
    acute hypercalcemia, 163
Lorazepam
    convulsive status epilepticus, 132
    critical care, 72
    propylene glycol content, 86
Low molecular weight heparin (LMWH)
    deep vein thrombosis, 50
    unstable angina and non ST elevation myocardial infarction, 35
Lugol's solution
    thyrotoxic crisis, 107

M

Macronutrients, 139
Maculopapular eruptions, 101
Magnesium
    acute hypercalcemia, 163
    acute hypomagnesemia, 167
    dosage, 16
    stable ventricular tachycardia, 9
Malignant hyperthermia, 82–83
Mannitol
    intracranial hypertension management, 62–63
Megaloblastic anemia, 120

Meropenem
>   intravenous dosage, 182
Metabolic acidosis
>   acute primary, 177–181
>   anion gap, 177
>   hyperchloremic (non-anion gap), 177–178
Methemoglobinemia, 120, 123–124
Methylene blue
>   methemoglobinemia, 124
Methylprednisolone
>   acute asthma exacerbations, 151
Metoclopramide
>   minimizing aspiration during enteral nutrition, 142
Metolazone
>   acute renal failure, 158
Metoprolol
>   ST-elevation myocardial infarction, 31
>   unstable angina and non-ST elevation myocardial infarction, 25
Mexiletine, 38
Midazolam
>   critical care, 71–72
>   refractive status epilepticus, 133–134
>   synchronized cardioversion algorithm for symptomatic
>   tachycardia management, 10
Milk of magnesia
>   acute hypomagnesemia, 167
Milrinone
>   acute decompensated heart failure, 36, 37
>   septic shock, 69
Mitral valve disease, 41
Modified National Institute of Health Stroke Scale, 59–60
Modified Ramsey Sedation Scale, 75
Moricizine, 38
Morphine
>   acute decompensated heart failure, 35, 37
>   critical care, 73
>   ST-elevation myocardial infarction, 33
>   unstable angina and non-ST elevation myocardial infarction, 27
MVI-12
>   propylene glycol content, 86
Myasthenia gravis
>   medications exacerbating weakness, 135

Myocardial infarction
    nonfatal
        short-term risk of, 22–23
    ST-elevation
        acute pharmacological management, 27–33
Myxedema coma, 107–108

N

N-acetylsteine (NAC)
    contrast-induced nephropathy prevention, 156
    ICU toxicological emergencies, 94
Nadolol
    variceal hemorrhage, 116
Naloxone
    ICU toxicological emergencies, 96–97
    minimizing aspiration during enteral nutrition, 142
Narrow complex stable supraventricular tachycardia
    amiodarone, 7, 8
    management, 7–8
National Institute of Health Stroke Scale, 59–60
Neomycin
    hepatic encephalopathy, 114
Nephritis, 159
Nephrogenic diabetes insipidus, 173
Nephropathy
    contrast-induced
        prevention, 155–156
    drug-induced
        obstructive, 160
Nesiritide
    acute decompensated heart failure, 36
Neuroleptic malignant syndrome, 147–148
Neurology, 131–135
Neuromuscular blockers
    factors altering effects, 82
    ICU, 79–80
    nondepolarizing, reversal, 81
Niacin
    ST-elevation myocardial infarction, 33
    unstable angina and non-ST elevation myocardial
        infarction, 27

Nicardipine
    acute cerebrovascular accident blood pressure
        management, 57
Nitroglycerin
    acute decompensated heart failure, 35, 37
    propylene glycol content, 86
    ST-elevation myocardial infarction, 31
    unstable angina and non-ST elevation myocardial
        infarction, 26
    variceal hemorrhage, 116
Nitroprusside
    acute cerebrovascular accident blood pressure manage-
        ment, 57
    acute decompensated heart failure, 36
Nizatidine
    stress-related mucosal damage prophylaxis, 88
Non-anion gap metabolic acidosis, 177–178
Nondepolarizing neuromuscular blockers
    reversal, 81
Non-ST elevation myocardial infarction, 23–24
Non-variceal upper gastrointestinal bleeding, 109–110
Norepinephrine
    acute decompensated heart failure, 36, 37
    anaphylaxis/anaphylactoid reactions, 20
    pulmonary embolism, 51
    septic shock, 67–68
Nutrient-drug interactions, 141
Nutrition, 137–142
    assessment, 137–139

O

Obstructive nephropathy, 160
Octreotide
    acute non-variceal upper gastrointestinal bleeding, 110
    ICU toxicological emergencies, 97
    variceal hemorrhage, 116
Olanzapine
    delirium, 74
Omeprazole
    stress-related mucosal damage prophylaxis, 88
Oxacillin
    intravenous dosage, 182

Oxygen therapy
    ST-elevation myocardial infarction, 33
    unstable angina and non-ST elevation myocardial
        infarction, 27

P

Packed red blood cell (PRBC)
    acute uremic bleeding, 159
    erythropoietin, critically ill patients, 83–85
Pamidronate
    acute hypercalcemia, 163
Pancreatitis, 118
Pancuronium, 79
Pantoprazole
    acute non-variceal upper gastrointestinal bleeding, 110
    stress-related mucosal damage prophylaxis, 88
    variceal hemorrhage, 116
Papillary necrosis, 160
Parenteral nutrition, 140–141
Penicillin
    intravenous dosage, 182
Pentobarbital
    intracranial hypertension management, 63
    propylene glycol content, 86
    refractive status epilepticus, 134
Pharmaceutical dosage forms
    that should not be crushed, 88
Phenobarbital
    convulsive status epilepticus, 133
    propylene glycol content, 86
    therapeutic drug monitoring in ICU, 92
Phenylephrine
    septic shock, 68
Phenytoin
    convulsive status epilepticus, 132–133
    interacting with nutrients, 141
    propylene glycol content, 86
    therapeutic drug monitoring in ICU, 92–93
Photosensitivity reactions, 101
Piperacillin
    intravenous dosage, 182
    VAP, 128

Pneumonia
    hospital-acquired
        management, 126–127
        prevention, 125–126
    ventilator-associated
        management, 126–127
        prevention, 125–126
Pneumonitis, 154
Potassium supplements
    acute hypercalcemia, 163
PRBC. *See* Packed red blood cell (PRBC)
Prednisone
    acute asthma exacerbations, 151
Pre-eclampsia, 47
Primary metabolic acidosis, 177–181
Procainamide, 38
    stable atrial fibrillation/atrial flutter, 6
    stable ventricular tachycardia, 8, 9
Propafenone, 38
    stable atrial fibrillation/atrial flutter, 6
Propofol
    critical care, 72
    refractive status epilepticus, 134
Propranolol
    ST-elevation myocardial infarction, 31
    thyrotoxic crisis, 107
    unstable angina and non-ST elevation myocardial infarction,
        25–26
    variceal hemorrhage, 116
Propylene glycol content
    of intravenous medications, 86
Propylthiouracil
    thyrotoxic crisis, 107
Prosthetic heart valves
    antithrombotic pharmacotherapy, 42
Protamine sulfate
    ICU toxicological emergencies, 97
Protein, 139
    daily needs, 138
Proton pump inhibitors
    acute non-variceal upper gastrointestinal bleeding, 110
Pseudorenal failure, 160

Psychiatric disorders, 143–149
Pulmonary, 149–154
Pulmonary disease, 154–155
Pulmonary embolism, 51
Pulmonary fibrosis, 154
Pulseless arrest algorithm
        ACLS, 1
Pulseless electrical activity
        algorithm, 3
        causes and management, 18–19
Pyridoxine
        refractive status epilepticus, 134

Q

Quinidine, 38

R

Rabeprazole
        stress-related mucosal damage prophylaxis, 88
Ramsey Sedation Scale, 75
Ranitidine
        stress-related mucosal damage prophylaxis, 88
Refractory ascites, 113
Renal, 155–160
Renal disease, 159–160
Renal failure, 47, 157
Renal replacement therapy
        continuous intravenous anti-infectives, 182
Reteplase (rPA)
        ST-elevation myocardial infarction, 28
Rheumatic mitral valve disease
        antithrombotic pharmacotherapy, 41
Right ventricular infarction, 34
Riker Sedation-Agitation Scale, 75–76
rPA. *See* Reteplase (rPA)

S

Sedation
        critical care, 71–72
Septic shock, 66–71
Serotonin syndrome, 145–147

Sevelamer
    hyperphosphatemia, 176
Severe sepsis, 66–71
Short-term risk of death or nonfatal myocardial infarction with
    unstable angina, 22–23
Skin discoloration, 102
Sodium bicarbonate
    acquired Torsades de Pointes, 44
    acute hyperkalemia, 165
    diabetic ketoacidosis, 104–105
    dosage, 16–17
    metabolic acidosis, 179
Sodium nitrite
    ICU toxicological emergencies, 98
Sodium nitroprusside
    ST-elevation myocardial infarction, 33
    unstable angina and non-ST elevation myocardial infarction, 27
Sodium polystyrene sulfonate
    acute hyperkalemia, 166
Sotalol, 39
    stable atrial fibrillation/atrial flutter, 6
    stable ventricular tachycardia, 8, 9
Spironolactone
    ascites, 112
    ST-elevation myocardial infarction, 32
Stable atrial fibrillation/atrial flutter, 5–7
Stable ventricular tachycardia (SVT)
    amiodarone, 12
    management, 8–9
Statins
    ST-elevation myocardial infarction, 32–33
    unstable angina and non-ST elevation myocardial infarction, 27
Steatonecrosis, 117
ST-elevation myocardial infarction
    acute pharmacological management, 27–33
Stevens-Johnson syndrome, 101
Streptokinase
    ST-elevation myocardial infarction, 28–29
Stress-related mucosal damage prophylaxis
    protocol, 88–90
Sulbactam
    intravenous dosage, 182

SVT. *See* Supra-ventricular tachycardia (SVT)
Synchronized cardioversion algorithm for symptomatic tachycardia
 management, 9–11
Systemic lupus erythematosis, 102

T

Tachycardia, 10
 algorithm, 4–5
  drug-induced, 160
 synchronized cardioversion algorithm for symptomatic, 9–11
Tazobactam
 intravenous dosage, 182
Tenecteplase (TNKase)
 ST-elevation myocardial infarction, 28
Tense ascites, 112–113
THAM. *See* Tromethamine (THAM)
Theophylline
 therapeutic drug monitoring in ICU, 93
Therapeutic drug monitoring
 ICU, 90–94
Thiamine
 convulsive status epilepticus, 132
Thrombocytopenia, 120
 heparin-induced, 121–122
Thrombolysis in myocardial infarction (TIMI)
 grade flows, 21
 risk score, 21–22
Thyrotoxic crisis, 106–107
TIMI. *See* Thrombolysis in myocardial infarction (TIMI)
Tinzaparin
 deep vein thrombosis, 50
 pulmonary embolism, 52
TNKase. *See* Tenecteplase (TNKase)
Tobramycin
 therapeutic drug monitoring in ICU, 93–94
Tocainide, 38
Torsades de Pointes, 43–44
Toxic epidermal necrolysis, 101
Toxicological emergency antidotes
 ICU, 94–99
tPA. *See* Alteplase (tPA)

Trimethoprim/sulfamethoxazole
        propylene glycol content, 86
Tromethamine (THAM)
        metabolic acidosis, 179–180

U

Unfractionated heparin
        ST-elevation myocardial infarction, 29
        unstable angina and non-ST elevation myocardial infarction,
                24–25
Unstable angina
        and non-ST elevation myocardial infarction
                acute pharmacological management, 23–24
                short-term risk of death or nonfatal myocardial infarction with,
                        22–23
Uremic bleeding, 159
Urticaria, 102

V

Valproic acid
        therapeutic drug monitoring in ICU, 94
Vancomycin
        intravenous dosage, 182
        therapeutic drug monitoring in ICU, 94
        VAP, 127
VAP. *See* Ventilator-associated pneumonia (VAP)
Variceal hemorrhage, 115–116
Vasopressin
        asystole algorithm, 3
        dosage, 17
        euvolemic hypernatremia, 173
        septic shock, 68
        variceal hemorrhage, 116
        ventricular fibrillation/pulseless ventricular tachycardia
                algorithm, 2
Vaughan Williams classification
        antiarrhythmics, 38–39
Venous thromboembolism prevention, 48–49
Ventilator-associated pneumonia (VAP)
        management, 126–127
        prevention, 125–126

Ventricular fibrillation/pulseless ventricular tachycardia algorithm, 2
Ventricular tachycardia, 8–9
Verapamil, 39
    dosage, 17
    stable atrial fibrillation/atrial flutter, 5
    ST-elevation myocardial infarction, 32
Vitamin B6 (pyridoxine)
    refractive status epilepticus, 134

W

Warfarin
    atrial fibrillation, 40
    elevated international normalized ratio, 52–54
    interacting with nutrients, 141
    prosthetic heart valves, 42
    pulmonary embolism, 51–52
    ST-elevation myocardial infarction, 30
Water deficit calculation, 174
Wide-complex tachycardia
    amiodarone, 12

Z

Zinc sulfate
    hepatic encephalopathy, 114
Zoledronate
    acute hypercalcemia, 163